MYCOBACTERIAL
SKIN
DISEASES

To the memory of my
Father and Mother
who encouraged me to study and
practise the art of medicine;
to my wife
Ina,
and our children
Cita, Reza, Eva, Nanda and Luky
who inspired and supported me
during the preparation of this book.

NEW CLINICAL APPLICATIONS

DERMATOLOGY

MYCOBACTERIAL SKIN DISEASES

Editor

MARWALI HARAHAP, MD

Professor of Dermatology
University of North Sumatra
Medical School, Rumah Sakit Pirngadi
Medan, Indonesia

KLUWER ACADEMIC PUBLISHERS
DORDRECHT / BOSTON / LONDON

Distributors

for the United States and Canada: Kluwer Academic Publishers, PO Box 358, Accord Station, Hingham, MA 02018-0358, USA
for all other countries: Kluwer Academic Publishers Group, Distribution Center, PO Box 322, 3300 AH Dordrecht, The Netherlands

British Library Cataloguing in Publication Data

Mycobacterial skin diseases.
1. Man. Skin. Mycobacterial diseases
I. Harahap, Marwali II. Series
616.5

ISBN 0–7462–0119–2
ISBN 0–85200–823–6 series

Copyright

Published in the United Kingdom by Kluwer Academic Publishers, PO Box 55, Lancaster, UK.

Kluwer Academic Publishers BV incorporates the publishing programmes of D. Reidel, Martinus Nijhoff, Dr W. Junk and MTP Press.

Printed in Great Britain by Butler & Tanner Ltd, Frome and London.

CONTENTS

Other titles in the *New Clinical Applications* Series:

Dermatology (Series Editor Dr J. L. Verbov)
Dermatological Surgery
Superficial Fungal Infections
Talking Points in Dermatology – I
Treatment in Dermatology
Current Concepts in Contact Dermatitis
Talking Points in Dermatology – II
Tumours, Lymphomas and Selected Paraproteinaemias
Relationships in Dermatology
Talking Points in Dermatology – III

Cardiology (Series Editor Dr D. Longmore)
Cardiology Screening

Rheumatology (Series Editors Dr J. J. Calabro and Dr W. Carson Dick)
Ankylosing Spondylitis
Infections and Arthritis
Osteoarthritis

Nephrology (Series Editor Dr G. R. D. Catto)
Continuous Ambulatory Peritoneal Dialysis
Management of Renal Hypertension
Chronic Renal Failure
Calculus Disease
Pregnancy and Renal Disorders
Multisystem Diseases
Glomerulonephritis I
Glomerulonephritis II
Haemodialysis
Transplantation

LIST OF AUTHORS

Jacinto Convit, MD
Director, Instituto de Biomedicina
Apartado 4043
Professor, Central University of Venezuela
Caracas 1010 A, Venezuela

John Michael Grange, MD, MSc
Reader in Clinical Microbiology
National Heart and Lung Institute
Dovehouse Street
London SW3 6LY
Honorary Consultant Clinical Microbiologist
National Heart and Chest Hospitals, London
Assistant Editor of *Tubercle*

Marwali Harahap, MD
Professor of Dermatology
University of North Sumatra Medical School, Rumah Sakit Pirngadi
Medan, Indonesia

A. Colin McDougall, MD, FRCP
Consultant in Clinical Research to the British Leprosy Relief Association (LEPRA)
Department of Dermatology
The Slade Hospital
Headington
Oxford OX3 7JH, England
Previously Leprosy Specialist Ministry of Health, Lusaka, Zambia, Africa and Medical Specialist, Queen Elisabeth Hospital, Aden, Federation of South Arabia

Kenneth Joseph Tomecki, MD
Staff Physician
Department of Dermatology
Cleveland Clinic Foundation
1 Clinic Center
Cleveland, OH 44195
USA

Marian Irene Ulrich, PhD
Head, Section of Immunology II
Instituto de Biomedicina
Apartado 4043
Aggregate Professor
Central University of Venezuela
Caracas 1010 A, Venezuela

GUEST EDITOR'S FOREWORD

We have endeavoured in this book to bring the reader up-to-date information, which will contribute to an enhanced ability to diagnose and treat mycobacterial skin diseases.

This volume is mainly concerned with conveying to dermatologists, microbiologists, immunologists, dermatologists in training, registrars in other specialties and interested family practitioners, a concise appraisal of some recent developments in the various aspects of mycobacterial skin diseases.

The chapters dealing with bacteriology, pathology and immunology have been planned to appear at the beginning of the book to provide the necessary conceptual framework for the section on clinical science, which deals with the variety of clinical states. The value of the clinical descriptions is vastly enhanced by a careful reading of the earlier chapters.

The contributing authors have been most cooperative in making this, the tenth volume in the *New Clinical Applications in Dermatology* series, an excellent treatise. I thank each of them for their superb contributions.

If this book stimulates and encourages a greater interest in, and a better understanding of, mycobacterial skin diseases, and enables physicians to serve more effectively those who suffer, the time and effort spent to produce it will be amply rewarded.

PROFESSOR MARWALI HARAHAP

SERIES EDITOR'S FOREWORD

It was with great pleasure that I heard of Professor Harahap's wish to produce a volume on mycobacterial skin diseases.

Both he himself and his chosen contributors are experts in the field of mycobacterial disease and they have combined to produce this important work which clearly merits a worldwide circulation and a readership encompassing many disciplines.

JULIAN VERBOV

ABOUT THE EDITORS

Dr Marwali Harahap, Professor of Dermatology at the University of North Sumatra School of Medicine, Medan, Indonesia, is guest editor for this special issue devoted to *Mycobacterial Skin Diseases*. He received his medical degree from the University of Indonesia, Jakarta. He was postgraduate fellow in dermatology at the University of California, San Francisco in 1964–66 and in plastic surgery at the Tokyo Women's Medical College, Tokyo in 1977.

Professional society affiliations include chairmanship of the Indonesian Society for Dermatovenereology, North Sumatra region, and Fellowship of the American Academy of Dermatology, the International Society of Dermatology: Tropical, Geographic and Ecologic, the International Society of Dermatologic Surgery, the International Leprosy Association and the Medical Society for the Study of Venereal Diseases. He holds honorary membership of the Philippine Dermatological Society.

He is the author of numerous publications in the *International Journal of Dermatology* and the *Journal of Dermatologic Surgery and Oncology*, some chapters in books, and is the Editor of two books: *Skin Surgery* and *Principles of Dermatologic Plastic Surgery*. He is now working on his forthcoming book on *Leg Ulcers*. He is also a member of the Honorary Editorial Board of *Medical Progress* and *Asean Journal of Clinical Sciences*.

Dr Julian Verbov is Consultant Dermatologist to Liverpool Health Authority and Honorary Clinical Lecturer in Dermatology at the University of Liverpool.

He is a member of the British Association of Dermatologists, representing the British Society for Paediatric Dermatology on its Executive Committee. He is Editor of the Proceedings of the North of England Dermatological Society. He is a Fellow of the Zoological Society of London and a Member of the Society of Authors. He is a popular national and international speaker and author of more than 210 publications.

His special interests include paediatric dermatology, inherited disorders, dermatoglyphics, pruritus ani, cutaneous polyarteritis nodosa, therapeutics, drug abuse and medical humour. He organizes the British Postgraduate Course in Paediatric Dermatology and is a Member of the Editorial Board of *Clinical and Experimental Dermatology*.

1

TUBERCULOSIS AND ENVIRONMENTAL (ATYPICAL) MYCOBACTERIOSES: BACTERIAL, PATHOLOGICAL AND IMMUNOLOGICAL ASPECTS

J. M. GRANGE

BACTERIOLOGY

For many centuries before the discovery of their causative agents, tuberculosis and leprosy were regarded as being transmissible diseases and in the 19th century tuberculosis of the skin became a well recognized occupational hazard of pathologists, anatomists and butchers[1]. The transmissible nature of tuberculosis was convincingly demonstrated in an extensive series of experiments on rabbits by Villemin in 1868, and in 1874 Hansen saw the leprosy bacillus in preparations of lesions of patients with lepromatous leprosy. In 1882 Robert Koch isolated the tubercle bacillus in pure culture from various forms of tuberculous lesions, induced the disease experimentally in animals and reisolated the bacilli from lesions in these animals, thereby fulfilling his well-known postulates for the establishment of the aetiology of an infectious disease.

Shortly afterwards, Ehrlich found that the tubercle and leprosy bacilli could be differentiated from other bacteria by the failure of dilute mineral acids to remove the coloration imparted by staining with an arylmethane dye. This property, acid-fastness, is still widely used to detect these bacilli in clinical material.

In 1896 Lehmann and Newmann assigned the tubercle and leprosy bacilli to the genus *Mycobacterium*. This name means 'fungus-bacterium' and owes its origin to the characteristic mould-like pellicle formed by *M. tuberculosis* when grown on liquid media. (The non-culturable leprosy bacillus was included in this genus on account of its acid-fastness.) The name *Mycobacterium* has, from time to time, led to the false assumption that members of this genus are more closely related to the fungi than other bacteria. In fact, the mycobacteria, although possessing several distinctive and distinguishing features, are true bacteria.

Towards the end of the 19th century, small but constant differences were found between tubercle bacilli from human and bovine sources and these bacilli were named *M. tuberculosis* var. *humanus* and var. *bovinus* respectively. Also, at that time, acid-fast bacilli were isolated from birds, cold-blooded animals (notably turtles and frogs) and from milk, butter, grasses, compost and other environmental sources. Although there were occasional reports of human disease due to these organisms, in general they received scant attention. An exception was the turtle tubercle bacillus (*M. chelonei*) which was isolated by Friedmann in 1903 and was used for many years as a vaccine for, and as an immunotherapeutic agent against, tuberculosis. Many individuals, inoculated intracutaneously with this bacillus, developed small, chronic, indurated abscesses at the inoculation site but the patients often welcomed this reaction as a sign that the remedy was working!

The classification of mycobacteria other than the tubercle and leprosy bacilli was, for several decades, in a state of chaos and they were therefore termed 'anonymous' mycobacteria. Other terms include 'atypical', 'tuberculoid', 'opportunist' and MOTT (Mycobacteria Other than Typical Tubercle) bacilli. A term now widely used is 'environmental mycobacteria' – a name that stresses that the majority of species in the genus *Mycobacterium* exist freely as environmental saprophytes. This view of the genus is usually obscured by the great attention paid to the major pathogens *M. tuberculosis* and *M. leprae*.

The environmental mycobacteria are particularly associated with water – wet soil, marshes, sphagnum bogs, lakes, streams, wells, rivers and estuaries[2]. Some species, such as *M. marinum* and *M. gordonae*, seem to prefer free water while others, such as *M. terrae,* prefer wet soil. Two species, *M. kansasii* and *M. xenopi,* have a particular tendency to colonize man-made water systems and have been isolated from water tanks, shower units and taps. Apparent outbreaks of mycobacterial disease in hospitals have been traced to the practice of rinsing specimen receptacles (sputum pots and urinals) in water contaminated by these bacilli.

Mycobacterium chelonei has also been isolated from water supplies and has, on more than one occasion, contaminated supposedly sterile materials for injection or for use during operative surgery. Cutaneous abscesses, singly or in small outbreaks, have followed the use of such contaminated materials (see below).

Being environmental saprophytes associated with water, exposure of man to these mycobacteria through drinking, bathing, showering and other aquatic activities is unavoidable. The extent of such exposure, and the species of mycobacteria to which individuals are exposed, inevitably varies from country to country and from region to region within a country. Clearly, such contact is not affected by public health measures designed to reduce the transmission of the major pathogens *M. tuberculosis* and *M. leprae* from person to person. There is ample evidence that repeated exposure to environmental mycobacteria has profound effects on immune reactivity. Such contact has been postulated as the cause of the widely varying results obtained in the major BCG trials, although opinions differ as to the exact mechanisms involved[3].

Although usually existing as harmless saprophytes, the environmental mycobacteria occasionally cause overt disease in the individuals whom they infect. Interest in this group of bacteria was awakened in the 1950s by the descriptions of two new cutaneous mycobacterial diseases; namely, *M. ulcerans* infection (Buruli ulcer) in Australia[4] and subsequently in Uganda and other tropical countries, and *M. marinum* infection (swimming pool granuloma) in Sweden[5]. This renewed interest led not only to the description of other forms of mycobacterial disease, including tuberculosis-like pulmonary disease, but also to serious attempts to classify the causative organisms. These studies were pioneered by Runyon[6] who introduced his well-known, though now somewhat obsolete, four-group classification; namely:

Group I	Photochromogens (pigment formed in the light)
Group II	Scotochromogens (pigment formed in the dark)
Group III	Non-chromogens
Group IV	Rapid growers

Following Runyon's work, extensive studies were conducted by the International Working Group on Mycobacterial Taxonomy (IWGMT) and, as a result, the genus *Mycobacterium* is now one of the best classified of all bacterial genera. The genus consists of about 50 known species, 41 of which are included in the Approved Lists of Bacterial Names[7] published in 1980 and several others have been described or reintroduced subsequently. These species are divided into three main groups: slow growers (Runyon's groups I–III), rapid growers (Runyon's group IV) and those that have never convincingly been cultivated *in vitro*.

About half the described species are frequent or rare causes of human disease: these are listed in Table 1.1. They include almost all the slowly growing species but only two of the rapid growers, namely, *M. chelonei* and *M. fortuitum*.

Many of the species listed in Table 1.1 cause disease that mimics the many clinical forms of tuberculosis but two species cause characteristic cutaneous lesions. These are *M. marinum,* the cause of swimming pool granuloma, also called fish tank granuloma and fish fancier's finger (Figure 1.1), and *M. ulcerans,* the cause of Buruli ulcer. Furthermore, with one exception, the few published reports of disease due to *M. haemophilum* have all been of granulomatous or ulcerative cutaneous lesions in immunosuppressed individuals.

Post-injection abscesses form a distinct and important class of the cutaneous mycobacterioses and are almost always due to the rapid growers *M. chelonei* and *M. fortuitum.* These were often grouped together as the 'Fortuitum complex', thereby concealing the fact that *M. chelonei* is the more virulent of the two. Both pathogens have long, interesting but rather confusing histories. They were first isolated in 1903 and 1905 respectively and belong to the group known as the 'cold-blooded tubercle bacilli'.

Mycobacterium chelonei was isolated from the sea turtle (*Chelona corticata*) and, as already mentioned, was used as a vaccine and therapeutic agent. Its synonyms include *M. abscessus, M. friedmanii*

TABLE 1.1 Causes of mycobacterial disease in man

(1)	Skin predominantly involved		
	M. leprae – leprosy		
	M. marinum (P) – swimming pool granuloma		
	M. ulcerans (N) – Buruli ulcer		
	M. haemophilum (N) – skin lesions in immunosuppressed individuals		
(2)	Major causes of post-injection abscesses and other post-traumatic lesions		
	M. chelonei (RG)		
	M. fortuitum (RG)		
(3)	Tuberculosis		
	M. tuberculosis		
	M. bovis		
	M. africanum		
(4)	Opportunist infection usually resembling tuberculosis (including occasional dermatological manifestations)		
	M. avium (N)	*M. scrofulaceum* (S)	*M. szulgai* (S)
	M. intracellulare (N)	*M. malmoense* (S)	*M. shimoidei* (N)
	M. kansasii (P)	*M. simiae* (P)	*M. terrae* (N)
	M. xenopi (N)	*M. asiaticum* (P)	
(5)	Infection caused by unidentified acid-fast bacilli. 'Feldman–Hershfield ulcers'		

P = Photochromogen; S = scotochromogen; N = non-chromogen; RG = rapid grower.

and *M. borstelense*. It has two distinct subtypes, *chelonei* and *abscessus*, which appear to be of equal virulence.

Mycobacterium fortuitum was isolated from the frog (*Rana temporaria*) and was named *M. ranae* but, owing to considerable confusion caused by mislabelled reference strains, the legitimate name was changed to *M. fortuitum*. Synonyms include *M. giae, M. minetti* and *M. peregrinum*. There are two main subtypes, *fortuitum* and *giae*, and nearly all disease is due to the first of these.

The slowly growing species are divisible into the '*M. tuberculosis* group' and the opportunist pathogens. The four members of the '*M. tuberculosis* group' are *M. tuberculosis* (the human tubercle bacillus), *M. bovis* (the bovine tubercle bacillus), *M. africanum* (a rather heterogeneous group of strains isolated originally from man in Equatorial Africa and which appear to bridge the gap between the human and

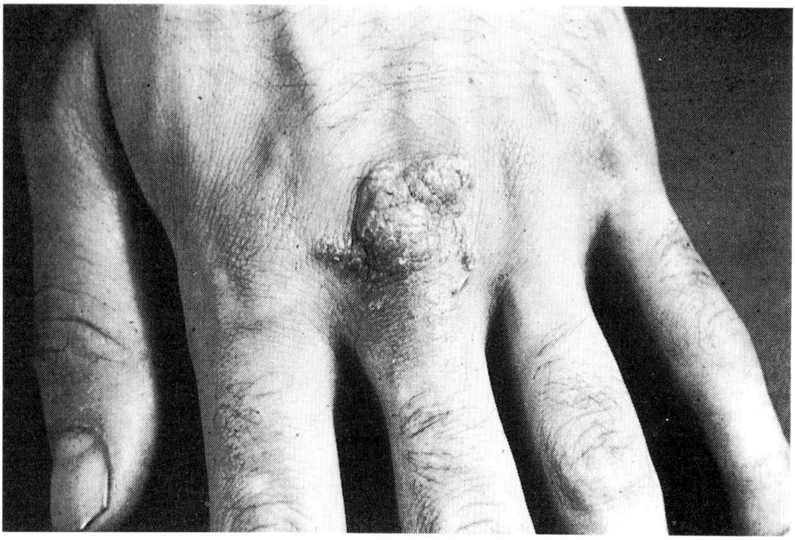

FIGURE 1.1 *Mycobacterium marinum* infection of the hand of a tropical fish keeper

bovine bacilli) and *M. microti* (the vole tubercle bacillus). The first three species cause all forms of tuberculosis in man and *M. microti* causes disease in voles and other small mammals but is attenuated for man. Indeed it was evaluated alongside BCG as a vaccine in man but, although its efficacy was equivalent to that of BCG, it was abandoned in favour of the latter as a small number of those vaccinated developed lupus vulgaris at the inoculation sites.

It must not be forgotten that the most prevalent cutaneous mycobacterial lesion encountered nowadays is that deliberately induced by BCG vaccination. Although almost always self-limiting, occasional abscesses occur, particularly when too much vaccine is given or it is injected too deep. Usually the diagnosis is obvious from the recent history of vaccination, although bacteriological confirmation is often sought. BCG was apparently derived from a bovine tubercle bacillus but it now has distinctive properties that permit its easy identification.

Most of the other slowly growing species cause disease in man and many cause cutaneous disease.

The two principal photochromogenic pathogens are *M. marinum* and *M. kansasii*. Although distinct species, they are very similar in their pigmentation and rate of growth. They often have elongated cells with a distinct banded or beaded appearance. Whereas *M. kansasii* grows well at 37°C, *M. marinum* grows very poorly, or not at all, at this temperature. Hence *M. marinum* infections are almost always limited to the skin but *M. kansasii* is more often associated with lung disease.

Pathogenic scotochromogens include *M. scrofulaceum* (the scrofula scotochromogen) which occasionally causes scrofuloderma and *M. szulgai* which has been reported as the cause of superficial bursitis and cutaneous granulomas.

The most important group of pathogens amongst the non-chromogens are *M. avium* (the avian tubercle bacillus) and *M. intracellulare*. These are so very closely related that they are often grouped together as *M. avium-intracellulare* or the MAI complex. They have attracted considerable interest recently as they often cause disseminated infections in patients with AIDS.

Two further non-chromogens of dermatological importance are *M. ulcerans*, a very slowly growing organism with a restricted temperature range of growth and *M. haemophilum*, an organism associated with skin lesions in immunosuppressed individuals and which requires high concentrations of haem or other iron sources for its growth. The other non-chromogens, listed in Table 1.1, only very rarely cause cutaneous disease in man. *Mycobacterium terrae* has been responsible for a few superficial infections acquired while farming or gardening[1].

A further group of mycobacteria requiring consideration are those that have never convincingly been cultivated *in vitro*. *Mycobacterium leprae* is the classical example and is discussed in Chapter 2 but others may also be involved in human cutaneous disease. In 1974 Feldman and Hershfield described an outbreak of skin ulcers containing non-culturable acid-fact bacilli occurring in non-immunosuppressed individuals living near the border of Canada and the USA[8]. Similar 'Feldman–Hershfield ulcers' have been seen in Brazil (H. L. David, personal communication).

Finally, a single case of skin ulceration due to a new mycobacterial species (subsequently termed *M. shinshuense*) has been described[9]. The patient, a 19-year-old Japanese girl, had an ulcer about 5 cm in diameter on the left elbow. Many acid-fast bacilli were seen in tissue biopsies and smears from the ulcer, which healed after 2 weeks of rifampicin therapy. The organism was of intermediate growth rate and grew at both 28 and 37°C, with much better growth at the lower temperature.

BACTERIOLOGICAL DIAGNOSIS

Isolation and identification of the causative organism is the principal diagnostic procedure in cutaneous mycobacterial disease, other than leprosy[10]. Biopsy specimens should always be collected into sterile containers in order to avoid contamination with environmentally-derived mycobacteria. When possible, specimens should be bisected, one being placed in fixative for histological examination and one, unfixed, for bacteriological investigations.

If the lesion is a pyogenic abscess, as may be caused by BCG, *M. chelonei, M. fortuitum* or *M. haemophilum*, it is better to send curettings or biopsies of the abscess wall rather than aspirated pus as the latter contains free fatty acids that may kill mycobacteria or inhibit their growth.

In the laboratory, tissues for microscopy and culture are homogenized by grinding (in a sterile Griffith tube or similar device) and smears are made from the homogenate for microscopy. Homogenates of clean specimens are inoculated directly on to media while those likely to be contaminated by other bacteria or fungi require chemical 'decontamination'.

Most of the culturable mycobacterial skin pathogens grow well on standard glycerol–egg media such as Löwenstein–Jensen (LJ) medium but *M. bovis* gives a feeble 'dysgonic' growth: much better growth of this species is obtained by substituting pyruvate for glycerol, as in Stonebrink's medium. *Mycobacterium haemophilum* requires an iron-supplemented medium such as LJ containing 2% ferric ammonium citrate (FAC).

Three species particularly associated with cutaneous disease, *M. marinum, M. ulcerans* and *M. haemophilum*, fail to grow at 37°C, particularly on primary isolation. Conversely, *M. chelonei* may grow at 37°C on primary isolation (perhaps as an adaptation to growth in the human host) but often fails to grow at this temperature on subculture.

Mycobacterium ulcerans has a particularly narrow temperature range of growth: 31–34°C.

Accordingly, when possible, skin homogenates should be inoculated on to two slopes each of LJ and LJ + FAC to be incubated at 32–33°C and at 35–37°C and one of pyruvate–egg medium for incubation at 35–37°C.

Members of the '*M. tuberculosis* group' are usually identified by their colony appearance, lack of pigmentation, failure to grow at 25°C and by a few simple biochemical tests. The identification of other mycobacteria is a skilled and specialized branch of microbiology and is usually undertaken by specialized reference laboratories.

MYCOBACTERIAL PROPERTIES OF RELEVANCE TO HUMAN DISEASE

Many of the distinctive characteristics of the mycobacteria, including their acid-fast staining properties, are associated with their very complex and lipid-rich cell walls. Furthermore, the peculiar structure of these cell walls probably accounts for many of the features of mycobacterial disease[11].

The mycobacterial cell wall is the most complex in all of nature. It consists of four main layers. The first, innermost, layer is composed of murein or peptidoglycan – a substance which, with minor variations, is found in all bacteria except the cell wall-free mycoplasmas. It consists of long polysaccharide chains cross-linked by shorter pentapeptide (five amino-acid) chains thereby forming a huge net-like macromolecule which gives the bacterial cell its shape and rigidity. In addition, the murein layer is largely responsible for the powerful adjuvant activity of the mycobacteria. Purified peptidoglycan induces granuloma formation in experimental animals.

The next layer is composed of arabinogalactan, a branched polysaccharide containing arabinose and galactose and also forming a net-like macromolecule. Attached to this structure are long-chain fatty acids termed mycolic acids. These contain about 80 carbon atoms, 60 or so in a long chain and about 20 in a single shorter branch. These fatty acids form the third layer – a dense pallisade which gives the cell its thickness, high lipid content and hydrophobic nature. The mycolic acids are responsible for acid-fastness and their synthesis is the target of the antituberculous drug isoniazid.

The fourth and outermost layer contains a complex group of substances collectively termed mycosides. These usually contain peptides, sugars and lipids and are analogous to the O antigens of the Gram-negative enteric bacteria. A related class of compounds are the phenolic glycolipids (PGL) and include PGL-1, an abundant surface component of *M. leprae*.

Mycosides are responsible for colony morphology, agglutination serotype and, in some cases, virulence. They are thought to contribute to the electron-transparent capsule-like structures surrounding some species of mycobacteria within macrophages and which may therefore have a protective function.

Other superficially situated sugar-containing lipids include trehalose dimycolate (cord factor) which was originally but erroneously thought to be responsible for the characteristic 'serpentine cords' seen in microcolonies of *M. tuberculosis*. The closely related sulpholipids are toxic and strongly acidic and, like cord factor, were thought to be major determinants of virulence, but this now appears unlikely.

A further important class of mycobacterial cell wall lipids consists of the arabinomannans (LAM). These are anchored to the cell membrane and extend through the cell wall to the surface. One of these, LAM-B, is an antigenically dominant molecule common to all mycobacteria.

Many publications, particularly older ones, refer to a substance termed wax D. This is a complex cell wall fragment, probably released in old cultures by autolysis, and consists of short segments of murein and arabinogalactan linked to a few mycolic acids. There is evidence that this substance is very stable and is not easily cleared from lesions. It may, therefore, particularly as it is a powerful adjuvant, be responsible for continuing 'disease', even in the absence (or virtual absence) of viable mycobacteria, as discussed below.

In addition to the mycosides and polysaccharide antigens referred to above, mycobacteria contain many soluble protein antigens, some of which are unique to each species and some of which are more widely shared[12]. Some antigens are only liberated on destruction of the bacterial cell but others are actively secreted by living cells. Mycobacterial antigens have been extensively studied for purposes of bacterial classification but very little is known of the contribution of individual antigens to the pathogenesis of, or immunity to, mycobacterial disease. The recent ability to obtain pure antigens in relatively large amounts by 'genetic engineering' should lead to exciting developments in this field.

CLASSIFICATION OF THE CUTANEOUS MYCOBACTERIOSES

Clinically, mycobacterial disease is divisible into that primarily involving the skin following traumatic inoculation of bacilli into the epidermis or dermis and that involving internal organs due, probably, to inhalation or ingestion of the bacilli. Cutaneous disease may occur as a secondary manifestation of the latter.

Many attempts have been made to classify the diverse forms of tuberculosis and other mycobacterioses of the skin but none has

TABLE 1.2 Classification of cutaneous disease due to *M. tuberculosis* and other cultivable mycobacteria

Primary lesions

(1) Inoculation into dermis or epidermis, e.g. primary cutaneous tuberculosis, *M. marinum* infection, Buruli ulcer

(2) Deeper inoculations, e.g. post-injection abscesses

Secondary lesions

(1) Inoculation into skin from endogenous source, e.g. from tuberculous sputum

(2) Lesions due to haematogenous dissemination

(3) Lesions due to lymphatic spread, e.g. 'sporotrichoid' lesions in *M. marinum* infection

(4) Lesions secondary to disease of underlying structures, e.g. scrofuloderma

Tertiary lesions

Lesions developing as a result of immunological phenomena rather than due to direct bacillary invasion, e.g. erythema nodosum

proved ideal. A suggested classification is shown in Table 1.2. The term 'primary' as used here implies that the cutaneous lesion develops at the site of the initial entry of the causative organism into the host, while the term 'secondary' is applied to lesions developing as a result of spread from a focus of disease elsewhere. Thus 'secondary' lesions may occur in disseminated primary disease and 'primary' cutaneous lesions may occur in tuberculin-positive (presumably previously infected) individuals. The latter type of lesions have been termed 'pseudo-primary complexes'. Thus inoculation tuberculosis ('prosector's wart') was probably often of this type during the last century when most adults had already been infected, whilst nowadays it is more likely to be a primary infection, particularly in countries where tuberculosis is now uncommon. The term 'tertiary' refers to a class of skin lesions that are generally not regarded as being directly due to the presence of viable mycobacteria.

IMMUNOPATHOLOGY

The immunological and histological features of mycobacterial disease are so intimately interwoven that they are best considered together.

Despite an enormous amount of research, the immunology of mycobacterial disease remains a challenging and complex subject with many unanswered questions. There are many gaps in our knowledge of the way in which mycobacteria are killed and eliminated, the role of the macrophage in this killing, the cause and nature of the characteristic delayed, necrotizing, cell-mediated (Type IV) hypersensitivity reaction and the relation of this to protective immunity.

A consideration of the cutaneous reactivity to mycobacterial antigens may usefully begin with an account of Robert Koch's[13] discovery of the delayed hypersensitivity reaction (later termed the Koch phenomenon) in the guinea pig. This account is best given in a translation of Koch's own words:

> 'When a healthy guinea pig is inoculated with a pure culture of tubercle bacilli, the inoculation wound usually closes and, for a few days, appears to heal. After 10–14 days, however, a hard nodule appears and soon breaks down to form an ulcer that remains until the animal dies. A totally different reaction ensues when a guinea pig which already has tuberculosis is challenged: this is best seen in animals given their first challenge 4–6 weeks previously. The small inoculation wound also closes initially in such

animals but no nodule is formed; instead, a characteristic change occurs at the inoculation site over the next day or two. The region becomes indurated and acquires a dusky colour which is not restricted to the point of inoculation but spreads into the surrounding skin up to a diameter of 0.5–1 centimetre. During the next few days the skin becomes overtly necrotic and eventually sloughs off, leaving a shallow ulcer which usually heals rapidly and permanently and does not lead to involvement of the neighbouring lymph nodes. Hence tubercle bacilli affect the skin of a healthy animal in a manner entirely different to that of a tuberculous one. This striking effect is not only elicited by living tubercle bacilli but also by dead ones, irrespective of whether they were killed by prolonged storage at low temperatures, as in my early investigations, or by boiling or by certain chemicals.'

Subsequently Koch obtained an identical reactivity by using a heat-concentrated filtrate of the medium in which tubercle bacilli had been grown – a preparation termed Old Tuberculin. Attempts to use this, and related, preparations for the treatment of tuberculosis were generally unsuccessful although there is considerable evidence that it was beneficial in some cases of chronic cutaneous tuberculosis (lupus vulgaris). Koch's work was, however, not in vain as the hypersensitivity reaction induced by Old Tuberculin in previously infected subjects became the basis of the tuberculin test. It also became the subject of a lengthy debate on its relevance to protective immunity – a debate that has still not been fully resolved.

CUTANEOUS REACTIVITY TO MYCOBACTERIAL ANTIGENS

As mentioned above, Koch found that the dermal reactivity induced in the sensitized guinea pig by Old Tuberculin was identical to that induced by viable and virulent tubercle bacilli. Thus the tuberculin test provides a convenient and clinically relevant way of studying the early events in the dermis following the introduction of mycobacteria.

The nature of tuberculin reactivity has been the subject of a number of studies undertaken at Airlangga University, Surabaya, Indonesia, by Kardjito and his colleagues. These workers have shown that there are at least three distinct elements to the positive tuberculin reaction: early erythema (6–24 hours), later firm induration (maximal between

48 and 72 hours) and an infiltration of the dermis by blood-borne white cells.

The erythematous reaction, read at 6–8 hours, is seen much more frequently in patients with active tuberculosis than in healthy tuberculin-positive individuals[14], although the distinction is not great enough to be of diagnostic value. More surprisingly, this early component of the tuberculin reaction is particularly frequent and extensive in hospital workers who are regularly exposed to patients with open tuberculosis and who are therefore, presumably, repeatedly reinfected. This phenomenon was observed in hospitals in both Indonesia and England[15,16].

The nature of the early erythematous reaction is unknown: its size does not correlate with serum levels of antibody of *M. tuberculosis* in the IgG, IgM, IgA or IgE immunoglobulin classes or in the four subclasses of IgG. It is therefore unlikely to be either a delayed atopic (Type I) or an immune complex-mediated (Arthus or Type III) hypersensitivity reaction. Whatever immune phenomenon it represents, it may be of great importance as a 'gatekeeper' reaction and may thus determine the nature of the subsequent immune reactivity at the inoculation site.

The cellular infiltration is seen around dermal capillaries and appendages (sweat glands and hair follicles) and is composed of blood-borne leukocytes. In addition to these discrete perivascular and periappendicular inflammatory foci, some mononuclear cells (lymphocytes and monocytes) migrate out into the interstitial dermis: these cells are particularly numerous in the subepidermal region (Figure 1.2). Although the focal inflammation is non-specific, the interstitial cellular infiltrate appears to be in response to the species-specific mycobacterial antigens. Biopsies taken from the centres of tuberculin test sites at 48 hours show that between 5 and 50% of the dermis is occupied by such focal cellular infiltrates yet, surprisingly, there is no correlation between the intensity of this inflammatory reaction and the extent of clinically evident induration. Indeed, some individuals with no visible or palpable induration have extensive focal cellular infiltrates[17].

Accordingly, and contrary to a widespread assumption, the induration seen in the tuberculin reaction is not directly due to the accumulation of cells at the test site. It is more likely to be due to oedema

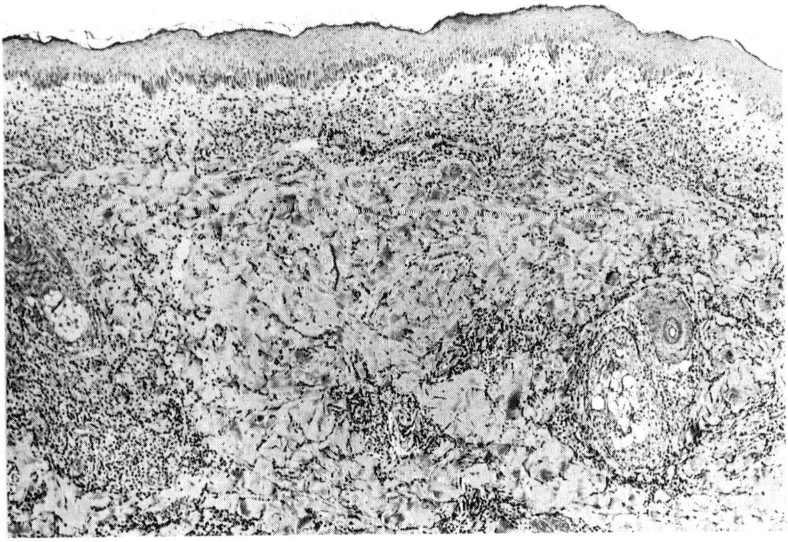

FIGURE 1.2 Histological section of a tuberculin reaction at 48 hours

which, in turn, is the result of changes in capillary permeability and blood flow rates due to vasoactive mediators released by cells in the perivascular foci.

The necrosis seen in many forms of postprimary tuberculosis and also in very severe tuberculin reactions may also be the result of vascular changes[18]. The increased cellularity at the site of infection or of a tuberculin test inevitably leads to an increased oxygen requirement of the tissue and a compensatory increase in the blood flow rate. Blood flow studies by laser Doppler velocimetry have shown that, in small to moderate-sized tuberculin reactions, the local blood flow rate increases more or less in proportion to the increased cellularity. In large reactions with signs of incipient necrosis there is an increase in blood flow rate at the edge of the induration but a considerable slowing in the centre. This reduction in blood flow relative to the cellularity is, in some cases, sufficient to predispose to ischaemia and subsequent tissue necrosis. The cause of the slowing of the blood flow rate is unknown but a possible candidate is tumour necrosis factor (TNF), as this affects vascular endothelium[19]. TNF is one of the mediators secreted by activated macrophages and is identical to cachectin, the substance thought to be largely responsible for the extreme wasting seen in advanced and untreated tuberculosis.

RELATION BETWEEN DELAYED HYPERSENSITIVITY AND PROTECTIVE CELL-MEDIATED IMMUNITY

There has been considerable debate for many years as to whether delayed hypersensitivity (DH) is an exaggerated but otherwise qualitatively identical form of the immune reaction responsible for protective cell-mediated immunity (CMI) or whether it is a distinct and dissociable reaction. The latter view has received support from Rook and Stanford[20] who have postulated that tuberculin reactions in mice may reflect either a protective macrophage-activating reaction similar to that induced by infection with *Listeria monocytogenes* or a hypersensitivity reaction analogous to the Koch phenomenon in guinea pigs. Thus the two reactions were termed the 'Listeria-type' and the 'Koch-type' respectively. It has also been claimed[21] that the two reactions occur in man and may be differentiated by their appearance at 48–72 hours. Reactions identified as 'Listeria-type' are pink, soft, rather ill-defined and tender but not painful on palpation. Those identified as 'Koch-type' have a well-defined, hard, purple-coloured area of induration with prominent hair follicles (peau d'orange) and occasional small bullae and they are painful on palpation.

An important point to note from Koch's original experiments on guinea pigs is that, although the altered dermal reactivity in infected animals enabled them to eliminate the bacilli introduced into the skin at the second challenge, the animals nevertheless eventually died of systemic tuberculosis induced by the primary challenge. From this it may be concluded that either this altered reactivity occurs in the skin but not in the deep tissues or that, if it occurs in the latter, it is non-protective or even antagonistic to protection in that situation.

It has already been stressed that tissue necrosis is a characteristic feature of delayed hypersensitivity. In the lung, such reactivity leads to extensive necrosis or caseation which is then liquefied by macrophage-derived proteases. When such a lesion erodes into a bronchus its liquefied contents are expelled and a cavity – the ideal breeding ground for tubercle bacilli – is formed.

Accordingly, the relevance of the necrotic component of the immune response to mycobacteria may be quite different when the infecting bacilli are in the skin, which is readily sloughed off when it becomes necrotic, than when they are embedded in the lung or other deep organ. In this respect it is noteworthy that strains of mice that are good 'Koch-type' reactors respond well to cutaneous challenge with *M. tuberculosis* but poorly to intravenous challenge, while the reverse is the case for mice that are principally 'Listeria-type' reactors. Furthermore, immunotherapeutic measures (tuberculin and vitamin D administration; see below) that have been shown to be of benefit in skin tuberculosis may facilitate the extension of the disease process in the lung. For a further understanding of this paradox it is necessary to consider the function of the macrophage in mycobacterial disease.

MACROPHAGE ACTIVATION AND GRANULOMA FORMATION

In the two decades since the classical studies of Mackaness[22] it has been widely accepted that macrophage activation is a cardinal feature of the immune reactivity and immunopathology of mycobacterial disease. In contrast to the short-lived polymorphonuclear leukocytes involved in acute inflammation and the early phase of cutaneous mycobacterial disease (see below), the macrophage is a long-lived cell involved principally in chronic infections. Macrophages are derived from blood and tissue monocytes and they develop certain characteristics depending on which tissue or organ they settle in. Although the intracellular killing of micro-organisms is a major function of macrophages, these cells are also secretors of a wide range of mediators, some of which are of central relevance to the immunological and pathological characteristics of mycobacterial disease.

For a full expression of their microbicidal and secretory properties, macrophages require activation, either non-specifically by bacterial adjuvants or specifically by antigens of the pathogen and the host's immune system.

The steps involved in the activation of macrophages are shown in Figure 1.3. Bacterial antigen is engulfed by cells known as antigen presenting cells (APC): these are thought to be derived from the same lineage of cells as those of the monocyte–macrophage series and

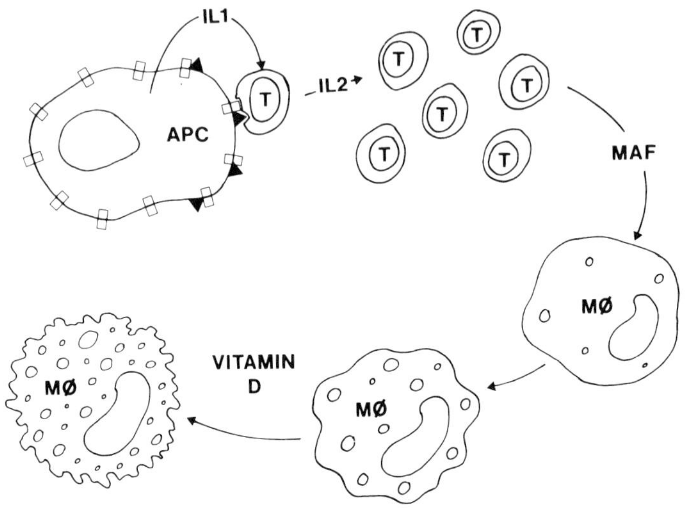

FIGURE 1.3 The steps involved in the activation of macrophages. For explanation see text. APC = antigen presenting cell; T = helper T-cell; MØ = macrophage, MAF- = macrophage activating factor

include the dendritic cells of lymphoid tissue and the Langerhans cells of the epidermis. These cells digest foreign proteins by means of enzymes in the cell membrane and individual antigenic determinants (epitopes) are 'presented' on the cell surface in close association with one of the cell's own surface antigens – the Ia (immune associated) antigen – coded for by the D region of the major histocompatibility complex. Lymphocytes of the T-helper-inducer (CD4) type with receptors specific for this host/foreign antigen complex bind to the APC and become activated. The exact mechanism of this lymphocyte activation is unclear but it involves a mediator, Interleukin 1, released by the APC. (In general, mediators liberated by cells of the immune system are termed lymphokines or monokines, depending on which class of cell releases them, but certain well characterized ones are termed interleukins.) The activated T-cell releases T-cell growth factor, Interleukin 2, which causes this and other T-cells bound to the APC to divide and produce a clone of identical cells. Clones of T-helper cells are able to activate macrophages by liberating a range of lymphokines collectively termed macrophage activating factor (MAF). The best known of these factors, though not necessarily the most relevant in mycobacterial disease, is gamma interferon (INF-γ). Activation of the macrophage causes its metabolism and oxygen consumption to increase. Its membrane becomes more motile, giving it a ruffled appearance, and its phagocytic and microbicidal powers are enhanced.

Treatment of human macrophages with lymphokines *in vitro* enables these cells to partially inhibit the growth of intracellular tubercle bacilli but, so far, actual killing of the bacilli has not been convincingly demonstrated. Treatment with INF-γ alone actually led to increased intracellular growth of tubercle bacilli in some experiments, but the inhibitory power of INF-γ treated macrophages could be enhanced by adding 1,25(OH)2-vitamin D3 to the culture medium. This may well explain the apparent therapeutic success of vitamin D, cod liver oil and ultra-violet light in the therapy of cutaneous tuberculosis[19].

The granuloma develops as a result of the attraction of monocytes to the site of chronic infection and their subsequent activation. Mature and activated macrophages are termed epithelioid cells and some of these fuse to form the characteristic multinucleate giant cells.

As already mentioned, activated macrophages secrete a wide range of substances. These include proteases and tumour necrosis factor, both of which almost certainly contribute to tissue necrosis and liquefaction of the necrotic material. In the case of the lung this necrotic process leads to cavity formation but the same process may cause the sloughing off of infected skin, as in Koch's original experiments. This is the likely explanation of the paradox of a reaction that eliminates tubercle bacilli from the skin of animals dying of systemic tuberculosis. It also explains why the administration of Old Tuberculin or vitamin D was apparently beneficial in cases of skin tuberculosis but sometimes led to an extension of pulmonary disease.

PERSISTING MYCOBACTERIAL DEBRIS AND DISEASE

It has been postulated that tuberculoid leprosy is largely the result of an exaggerated granulomatous response to mycobacterial fragments[19]. This might also explain some of the features of chronic cutaneous tuberculosis. Thus it has been shown that chronic granulomas may be induced by the injection of wax D into the skin of experimental animals and also that in BCG vaccination sites, wax D persists long after protein and polysaccharide mycobacterial antigens have been cleared from the vaccination site[23]. Not only is wax D difficult to eliminate but it is also a powerful macrophage-activating and granuloma-inducing adjuvant. Thus, there may well be similarities in the pathogenesis of the chronic paucibacillary form of cutaneous tuberculosis (lupus vulgaris) and tuberculoid leprosy, even though in other respects the immunological spectra in the two diseases may not be directly comparable. Both may be examples of what could be termed 'hyperactive' (as opposed to 'hypersensitive') granulomas.

THE IMMUNOLOGICAL SPECTRUM IN MYCOBACTERIAL DISEASE AND ITS RELEVANCE TO CUTANEOUS INFECTION

There have been several attempts to classify cases of tuberculosis into a spectrum of activity according to clinical and immunological features, but with rather limited success. In contrast to leprosy, such spectra were not defined histologically owing to the difficulty in obtaining tissue in all cases except cutaneous ones. Ridley and Ridley[24], however, were able to obtain biopsy material from 54 patients with tuberculosis and divided these according to their histological features into three groups, each with two subdivisions, as shown in Table 1.3.

Notably, all seven patients in Group 1 had cutaneous tuberculosis: either lupus vulgaris or solitary ulcerated lesions. Those in Group 2 (42 patients) had the common forms of tuberculosis affecting the lungs, lymph nodes and other internal organs, while the five patients in Group 3 had disseminated disease.

Although acid-fast bacilli were rarely seen in the Group 1 lesions, staining by the immunoperoxidase method revealed that the lesions contained diffusely distributed mycobacterial antigen within the macrophages and adherent to the connective tissue[25]. This antigen was particularly conspicuous in the perivascular regions of developing tubercles.

The question, as to whether the immunological spectrum of tuberculosis of the skin (and other tissues) is analogous to the spectrum of reactivity seen in leprosy, has often been raised[26]. Certainly most of the cutaneous lesions of patients in the study of Ridley and Ridley[24]

TABLE 1.3 Histological classification of tuberculosis. Data from Ridley and Ridley[24]

Group	*Main cell type*	*Type of necrosis*	*Giant cells*	*Bacilli*
1a	mature, organized epithelioid cells	none	+	none
1b	unorganized mature and immature epithelioid cells	patchy fibrinoid	+	rare
2a	immature epithelioid cells	caseation, no nuclear debris	+	occasional
2b	immature epithelioid cells or undifferentiated histiocytes	necrosis with nuclear debris and polymorphs	+	1–2+
3a	scanty macrophages	extensive, basophilic, coarse nuclear debris	–	2–3+
3b	very few macrophages	extensive, eosinophilic, not much nuclear debris	–	>3+

had some features in common with the lesions of tuberculoid leprosy; namely, well organized granulomas (tubercles) with mature epithelioid cells and giant cells, no or minimal necrosis and no detectable acid-fast bacilli. Patients with disseminated tuberculosis show a spectrum of immune reactivity from true miliary disease, with some degree of tubercle formation, to anergic cryptic disseminated disease with small necrotic lesions teeming with bacilli. The skin may be involved in disseminated tuberculosis and this has been termed tuberculosis cutis miliaris disseminata. These patients are almost always unreactive to tuberculin and are often extremely ill.

Immunologically unreactive tuberculosis and infections with other mycobacterial species may occur in immunosuppressed individuals, such as those on long-term steroid therapy, homograft recipients and victims of the acquired immune deficiency syndrome (AIDS). Such individuals, particularly those with AIDS, are very prone to tuberculosis and also to infection by *M. avium-intracellulare*; the histological features of the latter may closely resemble those of lepromatous leprosy (LL)[27]. This appearance is usually seen in individuals with disseminated disease but it has also been observed in more localized lesions. One patient, an asthmatic on long-term steroid therapy, had a papule 1 cm in diameter, on his forearm: the histological picture was compatible with LL but *M. avium* was isolated[28]. Excision of the lesion proved curative. Likewise, the Feldman–Hershfield ulcers had the histological features of LL.

Thus, polar forms of cutaneous mycobacterial disease similar to those seen in leprosy have been well described but there is no conclusive evidence for analogues of the intermediate or borderline forms of leprosy in the other mycobacterial diseases.

There may, however, be a stage in which there is some degree of cell-mediated immunity in the presence of a substantial bacterial load and this may lead to a mixed pyogenic and granulomatous picture – a condition termed suppurative granulomatous dermatitis[29]. This is seen in the early stages of primary inoculation tuberculosis and in lesions due to other mycobacterial species, except for post-injection abscesses and some deep lesions in immunosuppressed individuals which may be frankly pyogenic. Histologically there is a mixed picture of granulomas and abscesses: granulomas may contain either amorphous caseous material or numerous disintegrating polymorphs and many bacilli. This corresponds to Group 2b in the classification of Ridley and Ridley[24]. This suppurative component is seen in early lesions of swimming pool granuloma (*M. marinum* infection) and also in similar, but less common, superficial warty lesions due to *M. kansasii*[30] and *M. chelonei*[31], but after 4–6 months the histological picture of these infections is one of tuberculoid granulomas similar to those of lupus vulgaris.

A further class of cutaneous mycobacterial disease is that secondary to established disease of internal organs or structures. Two main types are seen: that in which sputum-derived bacilli are implanted into the skin (tuberculosis cutis orificialis) and skin disease due to direct extension of disease from an underlying lesion (scrofuloderma). The histological features of both differ from those of the other cutaneous mycobacterioses. Scrofuloderma is characterized by a necrotic abscess, ulcer or sinus track surrounded by caseating granulomas. Bacilli are usually seen. There may be associated lupus vulgaris in the more long-standing cases (Figure 1.4).

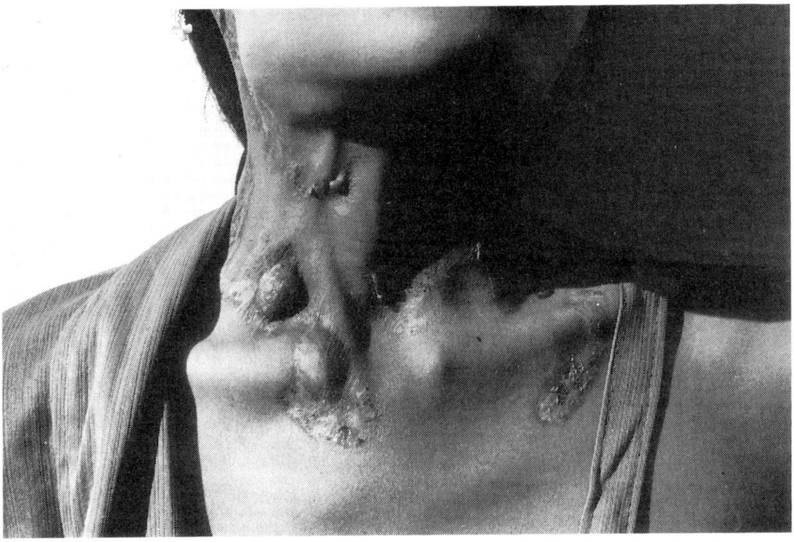

FIGURE 1.4 Scrofuloderma with secondary lupus vulgaris in a young Indonesian lady (courtesy Dr T. Kardjito)

Orificial lesions usually show non-specific inflammation and ulceration. Some reports claim that the tuberculin test is negative in patients with this rarely encountered form of tuberculosis: for reasons already discussed, a strong hypersensitivity reaction might prevent such cutaneous lesions from developing.

TRANSEPITHELIAL ELIMINATION OF TUBERCULOUS GRANULOMAS

Transepithelial elimination is a recently described phenomenon occurring in many skin disorders and may represent a normal mechanism for the skin to rid itself of infecting organisms and foreign bodies. One case involving skin tuberculosis has been reported[32]. Histological sections showed a distinct epithelialized transepidermal canal over a region of non-caseating tuberculous granulomas containing occasional acid-fast bacilli. The mechanism is unknown but it is distinct from the epidermal necrosis associated with anoxia and hypersensitivity.

SUMMARY OF HISTOLOGICAL FEATURES

Table 1.4, based on a number of useful reviews[29,33–35], summarizes the histological features of the major forms of cutaneous mycobacterial disease.

The pattern of reactivity is shown in Figure 1.5 which is based on a review of granulomatous inflammation by Adams[36]. After the initial acute inflammatory reaction (which is probably a non-specific response) there are four main possibilities, although the lesion may change from one form to another or two types may be present in the same patient or even in different parts of the same lesion. Chronic granulomatous inflammation may take many histological forms but two main patterns are seen: typical caseating tubercles associated with delayed hypersensitivity and, as in lupus vulgaris, a non-caseating granulomatous response to a minute, often undetectable bacterial load, i.e. a hyperactive state.

THE TUBERCULIDS

There is no area within the subject of cutaneous mycobacterial disease that is more mysterious than the motley collection of rashes and lesions grouped under the epithet 'tuberculids'. This name is usually applied to skin lesions that do not appear to be the result of direct invasion by viable acid-fast bacteria. Traditional explanations of their pathogenesis include reactions to mycobacterial 'toxins', violent hypersensitivity reactions to mycobacterial antigen (or whole bacilli) lodged in capillaries, infection by minute or cell-wall-free variants of mycobacteria or Arthus (Type III hypersensitivity) reactions due to excess antibody. None of these are more than hypotheses and one is forced to agree with Hirsh and Johnson[35] that 'a critical analysis reveals that the pathogenesis of the tuberculides is poorly understood'.

TABLE 1.4 Histological features of the principal types of cutaneous mycobacterioses

Type	*Tuberculin reactivity*	*Histology*	*Acid-fast bacilli*
Primary inoculation	−ve (early)	early: non-specific necrosis and ulceration with polymorphonuclear infiltrate	early: many
	+ve (late)	late: tubercle formation ±caseation	late: few
Secondary inoculation	+ve	verrucose hyperplasia of the epidermis; abscesses with polymorphonuclear cells in the upper dermis; tubercles with caseation in the mid-dermis. Moderate fibrosis	occasional
Lupus vulgaris	+ve	variable changes in the epidermis; diffuse cellular infiltrate in upper dermis; perivascular infiltrate in lower dermis; variable granuloma formation; little or no caseation; marked fibrosis	rarely seen
Scrofuloderma	+ve	ulcer, abscess or sinus track surrounded by caseating tubercles	moderate numbers
Tuberculosis cutis orificialis	−ve (or weak +ve)	non-specific ulceration	many
Cutaneous lesions in disseminated tuberculosis	−ve	non-specific necrosis	numerous

Owing to the rarity of these conditions, there have been very few detailed comparative studies.

It may be concluded from a survey of the literature that skin lesions termed tuberculides fall into three main divisions:

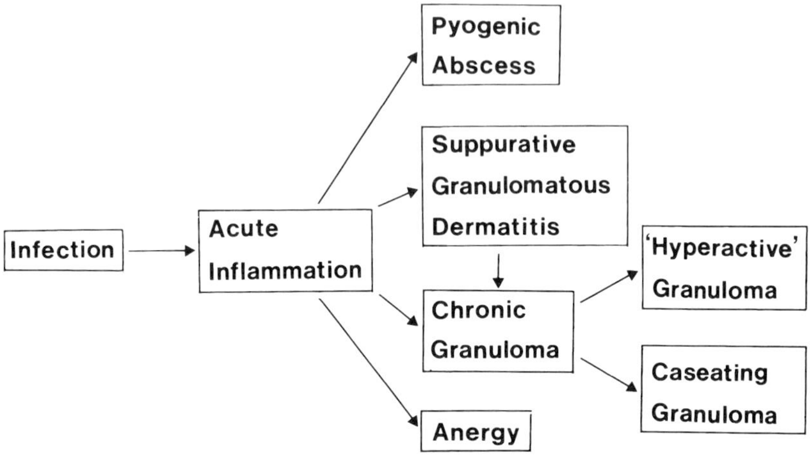

FIGURE 1.5 The pattern of immunological reactivity in cutaneous mycobacterioses

(1) nodular vasculitis – erythema nodosum and erythema induratum (Bazin's disease),

(2) 'true tuberculides', and

(3) lesions that histologically resemble those of tuberculosis but bear no direct association with that disease.

Erythema nodosum is a nodular vasculitis occurring in the subcutaneous adipose tissues. It is not specific to tuberculosis but occurs in several infectious diseases, notably streptococcal infections. Although rarely seen nowadays in the industrially developed nations, it was classically seen in children with primary tuberculosis at the time of onset of tuberculin reactivity and it was sometimes accompanied by fever and phlyctenular conjunctivitis. Erythema induratum is also a nodular vasculitis but it is more chronic than erythema nodosum and the lesions may progress to ulceration.

The 'true tuberculides' are discrete lesions that occur in patients with active tuberculosis or, rarely, disease due to other mycobacteria[37]. These tuberculides respond to antituberculous therapy, acid-fast bacilli have been seen in them and a minority of lesions progress to lupus vulgaris. Although there are many names for these lesions, two distinct types are recognizable: lichen scrofulosorum and papulonecrotic tuberculide[34]. The lesions occur in the dermis and differ with respect to necrosis. In lichen scrofulosorum there is a perivascular and periappendicular cell infiltration in the papillary dermis and granulomas with epithelioid and giant cells are seen but there is no caseous necrosis. Papulonecrotic tuberculides are similar but there is an obliterative vasculitis, probably the result of an Arthus or a delayed hypersensitivity reaction (or both), leading to necrosis[38]. In a minority of cases the necrosis is extensive and manifests as gangrene, and sometimes auto-amputation, of the extremities. Although individuals with either of these tuberculides are usually tuberculin-positive, there is no information on the qualitative nature of the tuberculin reaction. It would be fascinating to know whether those with lichen scrofulosorum gave the non-necrotic 'Listeria-type' reaction while those with papulonecrotic tuberculides gave the necrotizing 'Koch-type' reaction. There is evidence that those with the latter type of tuberculide are more strongly tuberculin-reactive than those with the former type[34].

The third group of lesions in this general category consists of those such as lupus miliaris disseminata which, despite a suggestive 'tuberculoid' histological appearance, have no proven relationship to tuberculosis. It is possible that these rare conditions are more related to sarcoidosis in their pathogenesis than to mycobacterial disease.

MYCOBACTERIUM ULCERANS INFECTION (BURULI ULCER)

This is a disease of such characteristic pathological and immunological features that it requires a separate consideration. There is strong epidemiological evidence that the bacillus is an environmental saprophyte that is inoculated into the skin by spiky or thorny plants or by other forms of injury. The first clinical feature is a small, indurated, painless but often itchy skin nodule mobile over the deeper tissues. In some individuals this primary lesion resolves but in others it increases in size and progresses to the ulcerative phase of the disease. This progression is characterized by a colliquative necrosis of the underlying adipose tissue down to the fascial sheath of the muscle. The overlying skin becomes anoxic and necrotic and eventually ulcerates with release of the liquefied necrotic fat and the formation of a characteristic deeply undermined ulcer. At this stage the lesion superficially resembles cavitating pulmonary tuberculosis and numerous acid-fast bacilli are found in the wall of the cavity underlying the skin ulcer. It also bears a resemblance to lepromatous leprosy as there is little or no histological evidence of a cellular immune response in the affected tissues. The patients fail to react to tuberculin and to Burulin, a specific skin-testing reagent prepared from *M. ulcerans*[39]. This pathological process leads to a progressive lesion with one or several ulcers. The lesion may be very extensive, sometimes involving a whole limb or the entire abdominal wall (Figure 1.6).

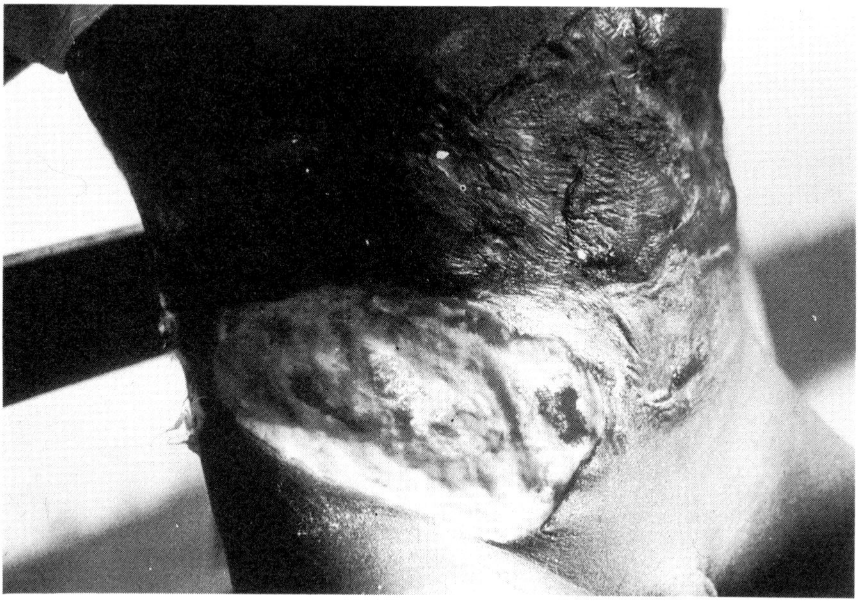

FIGURE 1.6 *Mycobacterium ulcerans* infection (Buruli ulcer) of the anterior abdominal wall of a Ghanaian boy (courtesy Dr A. Knell, Wellcome Tropical Institute)

The mechanism of the necrosis in *M. ulcerans* infection is uncertain but there is evidence that it is, at least in part, due to a bacterial exotoxin which has been identified as a high molecular weight phospholipoprotein–polysaccharide complex. This, when inoculated into the skin of a guinea pig, causes necrosis similar to that seen in the human lesions[40].

In virtually all cases, however, the disease process is self-limiting. A point is reached when, for unknown reasons, anergy is replaced by immunological reactivity, the patient becomes tuberculin- and Burulin-positive, there is a cellular infiltration with granuloma formation in the lesion, the bacilli diminish in number and then disappear. The lesion then heals, though often with gross and crippling deformities.

The cause and nature of the development of the immunological anergy and its subsequent reversal remain matters for speculation, although clearly their elucidation would have profound implications for the therapy of this uncommon but terrible mycobacterial disease, and possibly for others. One suggested cause of the anergy is the sequestration of specific lymphocytes in the lymph nodes.

Some patients with Buruli ulcer develop, for unknown reasons, extensive oedema of the affected region. The author saw a boy in Zaire with an ulcer about 12 cm in diameter on the thigh and gross oedema involving the whole limb. The oedema resolved after a few days of treatment with rifampicin, suggesting that it might be induced by a metabolic product of the bacillus. Mice infected with *M. ulcerans* frequently develop generalized oedema (the 'fat mouse syndrome') but it is not known whether this has the same cause as the oedema seen in man.

CONCLUSIONS

The bacteriological, immunological and pathological aspects of the cutaneous mycobacterioses remain challenging and complex topics. The diseases themselves continue to pose serious diagnostic and therapeutic challenges to the dermatologist. The diseases may be disfiguring, crippling and even life-threatening. While the classical forms of skin tuberculosis – lupus vulgaris and scrofuloderma – are rarities in the industrially developed nations, opportunist infections associated with immunodeficiency are encountered with increasing frequency. Inoculation mycobacterioses remain a worldwide problem[1] and take numerous forms, some mundane, some bizarre and some even comical as, for example, a 'brawl chancre' of the knuckle acquired by punching a tuberculous subject in the teeth! Others, notably Buruli ulcer, are tragic, often causing horrific mutilations.

Although most studies on tuberculosis focus on the pulmonary form of the disease, cutaneous manifestations offer an opportunity to look directly at the disease process, as may be done in leprosy. Indeed, a detailed cooperative comparative study of skin tuberculosis, leprosy and other cutaneous mycobacterioses might well open a treasure chest of information that would lead to major advances in the diagnosis, therapy and prevention of this group of human afflictions.

REFERENCES

1. Grange, J. M., Noble, W. C., Yates, M. D. and Collins, C. H. (1988). Inoculation mycobacterioses. *Clin. Exp. Dermatol*, **13,** 211–220
2. Collins, C. H., Grange, J. M. and Yates, M. D. (1984). Mycobacteria in water. *J. Appl. Bacteriol.*, **57,** 193–211
3. Grange, J. M. (1986). Environmental mycobacteria and BCG vaccination. *Tubercle*, **67,** 1–4
4. MacCallum, P., Tolhurst, J. C., Buckle, C. and Simmons, H. A. (1948). A new mycobacterial infection in man. *J. Pathol. Bacteriol.*, **60,** 93–122
5. Linell, F. and Norden, A. (1954). *Mycobacterium balnei:* a new acid-fast bacillus occurring in swimming pools and capable of producing skin lesions in humans. *Acta Tuberc. Scand.*, Suppl., **33,** 1–84
6. Runyon, E. H. (1959). Anonymous mycobacteria in pulmonary disease. *Med. Clin. N. Am.*, **43,** 273–90
7. Skerman, V. D. B., McGowan, V. and Sneath, P. H. A. (1980). Approved lists of bacterial names. *Int. J. Syst. Bacteriol.*, **30,** 225–420
8. Feldman, R. A. and Hershfield, E. (1974). Mycobacterial skin infections by an unidentified species: a report of 29 patients. *Ann. Intern. Med.*, **80,** 445–52
9. Tsukamura, M. and Mikoshiba, H. (1982). A new *Mycobacterium* which caused skin infection. *Microbiol. Immunol.*, **26,** 951–5
10. Collins, C. H., Grange, J. M. and Yates, M. D. (1985). *The Organization and Practice of Tuberculosis Bacteriology*. (London: Butterworths)
11. Grange, J. M. (1988). *Mycobacteria and Human Disease*. (London: Edward Arnold)
12. Stanford, J. L. and Grange, J. M. (1974). The meaning and structure of species as applied to mycobacteria. *Tubercle*, **55,** 143–52
13. Koch, R. (1891). Fortsetzung der Mitteilungen uber ein Heilmittel gegen Tuberculose. *Dtsch. Med. Wschr.*, **17,** 101–2
14. Kardjito, T. and Grange, J. M. (1982). Diagnosis of active tuberculosis by immunological methods. 2. Qualitative differences in the dermal response to tuberculin in patients with active pulmonary disease and healthy tuberculin-positive individuals. *Tubercle*, **63,** 275–8
15. Elansary, E. H. and Grange, J. M. (1984). Qualitative differences in tuberculin reactivity in patients with tuberculosis, occupational contacts and non-contacts. *Tubercle*, **65,** 191–4
16. Grange, J. M., Beck, J. S., Harper, E. I., Kardjito, T. and Stanford, J. L. (1986). The effect of occupational exposure to patients with tuberculosis on dermal

reactivity to four new tuberculins among healthy Indonesian adults. *Tubercle,* **67,** 109–18

17. Beck, J. S., Morley, S. M., Gibbs, J. H., Potts, R. C., Ilias, M. I., Kardjito, T., Grange, J. M., Stanford, J. L. and Brown, R. C. (1986). The cellular responses of tuberculosis and leprosy patients and of healthy controls in skin tests to new tuberculin and leprosin A. *Clin. Exp. Immunol.,* **64,** 484–94
18. Beck, J. S., Gibbs, J. H., Potts, R. C., Jawad, E. S., Kardjito, T., Spence, V. A. and Grange, J. M. (1989). The relation between cutaneous blood flow and cell content in the tuberculin reaction. *Scand. J. Immunol.,* **28,** in press
19. Rook, G. A. W. (1987). Progress in the immunology of the mycobacterioses. *Clin. Exp. Immunol.,* **69,** 1–9
20. Rook, G. A. W. and Stanford, J. L. (1979). The relevance to protection of three forms of delayed skin-test response evoked by *M. leprae* and other mycobacteria in mice. Correlation with the classical work in the guinea-pig. *Parasite Immunol.,* **1,** 111–23
21. Stanford, J. L. and Lema, E. (1983). The use of an ultrasonicate preparation of *Mycobacterium tuberculosis* (new tuberculin) in the assessment of BCG vaccination. *Tubercle,* **64,** 275–82
22. Mackaness, G. B. (1967). The immunology of antituberculous immunity. *Am. Rev. Respir. Dis.,* **97,** 337–44
23. Higuchi, S., Suga, M., Dannenberg, A. M., Affronti, L. F., Azuma, I., Daniel, T. M. and Petruli, J. P. (1981). Persistence of protein, carbohydrate and wax components of tubercle bacilli in dermal lesions. *Am. Rev. Respir. Dis.,* **123,** 397–401
24. Ridley, D. S. and Ridley, M. J. (1987). Rationale for the histological spectrum of tuberculosis. A basis for classification. *Pathology,* **19,** 186–92
25. Ridley, M. J. and Ridley, D. S. (1986). Histological demonstration of mycobacterial antigen, specific antibody and complement in the lesions of tuberculosis. *Histochem. J.,* **18,** 551–6
26. Skinsnes, O. K. (1968). Comparative pathogenesis of mycobacterioses. *Ann. N.Y. Acad. Sci.,* **154,** 19–31
27. Sohn, C. C., Schroff, R. W., Kliewer, K. E., Lebel, D. M. and Fligiels, S. (1983). Disseminated *Mycobacterium avium-intracellulare* infection in homosexual men with acquired cell-mediated immunodeficiency: a histologic and immunologic study of two cases. *Am. J. Clin. Pathol.,* **79,** 247–52
28. Cole, G. W. and Gebhard, J. (1979). *Mycobacterium avium* infection of the skin resembling lepromatous leprosy. *Br. J. Dermatol.,* **101,** 71–4
29. Savin, J. A. and Wilkinson, D. S. (1986). Mycobacterial infections including tuberculosis. In Rook, A., Wilkinson, D. S., Ebling, F. J. G., Champion, R. H. and Burton, J. L. (eds.) *Textbook of Dermatology.* pp. 791–822. (Oxford: Blackwell)
30. Hirsh, F. S. and Saffold, O. E. (1976). *Mycobacterium kansasii* infection with dermatologic manifestations. *Arch. Dermatol.,* **112,** 706–8
31. Yip, S. Y., Wu, P. C., Chan, W. C. and Teoh-Chan, C. H. (1979). Tuberculoid cutaneous infection due to a niacin-positive *Mycobacterium chelonei. Br. J. Dermatol.,* **101,** 63–9
32. Goette, D. K. and Odom, R. B. (1986). Transepithelial elimination of granulomas in cutaneous tuberculosis and sarcoidosis. *J. Am. Acad. Dermatol.,* **14,** 127–9
33. Brown, F. S., Anderson, R. H. and Burnett, J. W. (1982). Cutaneous tuberculosis. *J. Am. Acad. Dermatol.,* **6,** 101–6

34. Harahap, M. (1983). Tuberculosis and the skin. *Int. J. Dermatol.*, **22,** 542–5
35. Hirsh, B. C. and Johnson, W. C. (1984). Pathology of granulomatous disease. Epithelioid granulomas, part 1. *Int. J. Dermatol.*, **23,** 237–46
36. Adams, D. O. (1976). The granulomatous inflammatory response: a review. *Am. J. Pathol.*, **84,** 164–91
37. Grange, J. M. (1982). Mycobacteria and the skin. *Int. J. Dermatol.*, **21,** 497–503
38. Morrison, J. G. L. and Fourie, E. D. (1974). The papulonecrotic tuberculide – from Arthus reaction to lupus vulgaris. *Br. J. Dermatol.*, **91,** 263–70
39. Stanford, J. L., Revill, W. D. L., Gunthorpe, W. J. and Grange, J. M. (1975). The production and preliminary investigation of Burulin, a new skin test reagent for *Mycobacterium ulcerans* infection. *J. Hyg., Camb.*, **74,** 7–16
40. Hockmeyer, W. T., Krieg, R. E., Reich, M. and Johnson, R. D. (1978). Further characterization of *Mycobacterium ulcerans* toxin. *Infect. Immun.*, **21,** 124–8

2

LEPROSY: BACTERIAL, PATHOLOGICAL, IMMUNOLOGICAL AND IMMUNOPATHOLOGICAL ASPECTS

J. CONVIT and M. I. ULRICH

THE BACTERIOLOGY OF *MYCOBACTERIUM LEPRAE*

Introduction

Mycobacterium leprae is recognized historically as the first pathogenic bacterium visualized in infected human tissues, as reported by the Norwegian physician Armauer Hansen in 1874. In spite of innumerable efforts to cultivate this micro-organism *in vitro* and occasional unconfirmed reports of success, it remains as the only human pathogenic bacterium which has not been successfully cultured in artificial media. Koch's postulates for establishing the aetiological agents of infectious diseases have never been fulfilled in leprosy, but *M. leprae* is almost universally recognized as the causative agent of all clinical forms of the disease. Other micro-organisms, including mycobacteria of the avium–intracellulare–scrofulaceum complexes and leprosy-derived corynebacteria have been isolated from the lesions of leprosy with some regularity, but there is no convincing evidence that they contribute to the pathology of the disease or that they represent developmental stages in the life cycle of *M. leprae*.

The development of experimental animal models for studying *M. leprae* also presented an enormous challenge to investigators for nearly a century after its visualization in human tissues. The pioneering studies of Shepard, who reported limited multiplication in the normal mouse footpad in 1960[1] and of Rees, who achieved more extensive growth in irradiated, thymectomized mice[2], were followed by the demonstration of massive systemic infection of experimentally infected nine-banded armadillos by Kirchheimer and Storrs in 1971[3]. More recently, other experimental models including athymic mice and rats have expanded the repertoire of animal models of the disease. Many of the more recent bacteriological studies of *M. leprae* were made possible only when experimental infections in animals provided relatively large numbers of micro-organisms for study. The nine-banded armadillo represents the principal source of *M. leprae* for investigation at present, in spite of the difficulties associated with its maintenance in captivity.

Bacteriological classification and characteristics of *M. leprae*

M. leprae shares the morphological characteristics of other acid-fast mycobacteria when stained in tissue sections, and is taxonomically classified in the Order Actinomycetales and the Family Mycobacteriaceae, Genus *Mycobacterium*[4]. The individual bacilli, 0.3 μm in diameter and several microns in length, are slender, Gram-positive, acid-fast rods, which may be seen individually or in clumps of various sizes, including large irregular masses known as globi (Figures 2.1 and 2.2). Even in active untreated lesions, most organisms show an irregular staining pattern. *M. leprae* possesses at least five well defined distinctive properties which are widely recognized as criteria for its identification (Table 2.1).

(1) It is an obligate intracellular parasite which cannot be cultivated in artificial media.

(2) The acid-fast property of *M. leprae*, but not of other mycobacteria, is extractable with pyridine[5,6].

(3) *M. leprae* is the only mycobacterium that oxidizes D-dihydroxyphenylalanine (D-DOPA)[7].

(4) It is the only species of *Mycobacterium* which invades and grows within peripheral nerves.

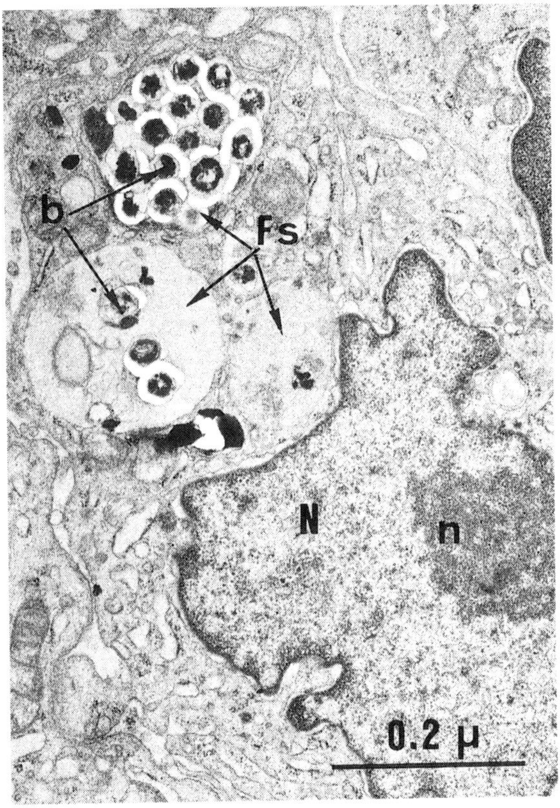

FIGURE 2.1 Electron micrograph of a transverse section of an infected macrophage from lepromatous leprosy, showing numerous bacilli (b) within foamy structures (Fs). N = nucleus; n = nucleolus. Original magnification × 13 000. Photo courtesy Dr A Bretaña

(5) Soluble extracts and whole bacillary preparations of *M. leprae* contain heat-stable antigenic components with characteristic immunological activity, inducing positive skin tests in patients with tuberculoid leprosy and negative reactions in lepromatous patients.

Most clinical centres are not equipped to demonstrate all of the characteristics of *M. leprae* described above, and usually such detailed analyses are not required. While the examination of histological sections is necessary for precise classification of leprosy, preliminary

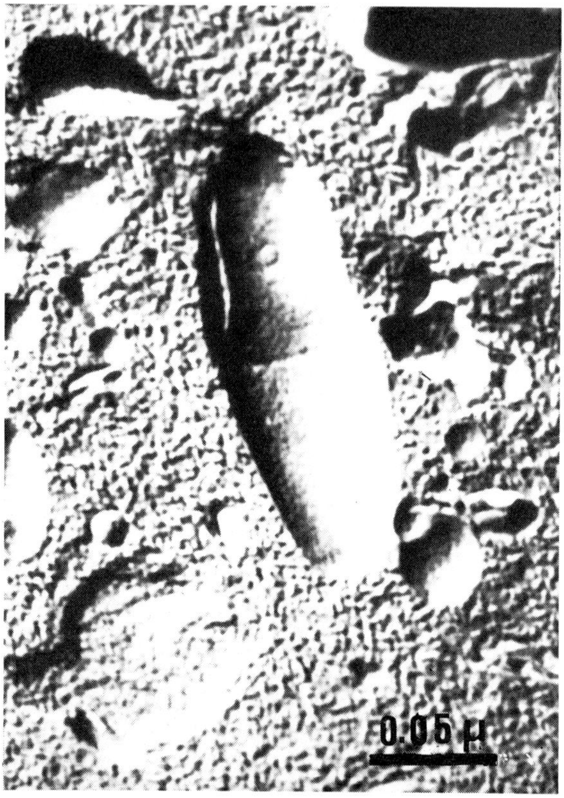

FIGURE 2.2 Detail of cell wall surface of *M. leprae* in a freeze-etching preparation. Original magnification × 35 000. Photo courtesy Dr A. Bretaña

diagnosis of the disease is usually made on the basis of clinical manifestations and the demonstration of acid-fast bacilli in slit-skin smears. This technique, described in detail elsewhere[8], consists of the staining of scrapings from a superficial cut in a small ischaemic fold of skin from the lesion, using the Ziehl–Neelson technique for staining acid-fast bacteria. In multibacillary disease, material from distant sites is also often examined. Ear lobes, elbows and knees are the most frequently examined distant sites, because of the predilection of *M. leprae* for relatively cool areas of the body surface.

TABLE 2.1 Primary distinguishing characteristics of *Mycobacterium leprae*

(1)	Acid-fast bacilli, obligate intracellular parasites non-cultivable in artificial media
(2)	Acid-fastness extractable with pyridine
(3)	Bacilli oxidize D-DOPA
(4)	Growth in Schwann cells and other nerve structures
(5)	Distinctive immunological activity in leprosy patients with polar forms of the disease

Bacteriological and morphological indices

Disease classification and evaluation of the efficacy of therapy, as well as other aspects of disease activity in leprosy, are often facilitated by the use of bacteriological and morphological indices, which permit a degree of quantification of the bacillary load and viability, in spite of the inability to cultivate *M. leprae in vitro*.

The bacteriological index (BI) is based on the enumeration of acid-fast bacilli in slit-skin smears, based on a logarithmic scale from 1+ (1–10 micro-organisms in 100 microscopic fields) to 6+ (>1000 bacilli per field)[9]. While this technique requires attention to technical details in smear preparation and staining, it provides a useful approximation of the relative mycobacterial population in lesions as well as at distant sites. The BI is of limited use in paucibacillary leprosy, but offers a useful tool in the evaluation of new cases of disease and of disease activity during the course of treatment.

The use of the morphological index (MI) is based on considerable clinical, microscopic and experimental evidence that viable *M. leprae* stain in a uniform manner, with even, intact borders; fragmented, beaded or irregularly staining bacteria are presumably dead[10,11]. Based on the examination of 100 acid-fast micro-organisms (when possible) in slit-skin smears stained under carefully controlled conditions, this index offers a useful guide in the evaluation of infectivity, response to therapy and detection of relapses or the possible development of drug resistance. Interestingly enough, the MI in untreated, active lesions rarely exceeds 5–10% of the total number of acid-fast bacilli; bactericidal drugs such as rifampin reduce the proportion of solid-staining mycobacteria very rapidly.

Biological characteristics of *M. leprae*

The reported generation time for *M. leprae* in normal and irradiated, thymectomized mice is 11–13 days[12,13]. This extraordinarily slow growth rate is undoubtedly the principal factor contributing to the exceptionally long incubation period, probably averaging 5–7 years, of lepromatous leprosy and to the chronicity of the disease in all of its clinical manifestations. This important question apparently has not been studied in the highly susceptible armadillo, which may develop massive fatal disease in less than 2 years. Interpretation of generation time data is complicated by the large numbers of non-viable mycobacteria in lesions; it has been suggested that the failure to consider the rapid death of many micro-organisms may contribute to a significant over-estimation of the generation time.

In addition to its unquestionably slow multiplication, *M. leprae* also demonstrates an extraordinary capacity to persist in a dormant viable state in the presence of bacteriostatic drugs such as Dapsone (DDS), so that monotherapy must be continued throughout the lifetime of multibacillary patients, even when they show no signs of clinical activity and skin smears are repeatedly negative. Whether multidrug therapy, which includes the use of bactericidal drugs, will alter this situation remains to be seen.

Considering the centuries-long clinical history of leprosy, it is quite remarkable that very few strain differences have been reported in isolates of *M. leprae* from many areas of the world. Shepard[14] has documented two stable types of limited growth of *M. leprae* in the footpads of normal mice, characterized by differing rates of growth and maximum plateau levels, but the two types are not associated with different forms of leprosy. More recently, strains showing resistance to DDS, rifampin and other drugs have been isolated with some frequency. Apparently no strain differences have as yet been demonstrated by biochemical or immunological criteria. These observations, coupled with the failure to grow *M. leprae in vitro* in spite of innumerable attempts and the very limited host range of natural infection, would suggest an extraordinarily intimate and restrictive relationship between the bacilli and host cells, severely limiting the possibility of survival of mutant forms of *M. leprae*.

The only known natural hosts of *M. leprae* are man and nine-banded armadillos[15]. Extremely rare natural occurrence in primates has been well documented.

Chemical and biochemical properties of *M. leprae*

Recent studies of *M. leprae* from experimentally infected armadillos have permitted detailed analyses of the chemical composition of these bacilli. While these studies will not be reviewed in detail, some of the more relevant observations will be briefly mentioned. Phenolic glycolipid I (PGL-I), described by Brennan and Barrow[16], is perhaps of particular interest to many field workers, since the native compound as well as synthetic neoglycoproteins bearing the same carbohydrate moieties possess highly specific serological activity. The serological tests based on the use of PGL-I or the synthetic antigens do not appear to be sufficiently sensitive to detect many paucibacillary or subclinical infections. Nevertheless, these tests are useful in highly selected healthy populations, such as the household contacts of lepromatous patients, as well as in the evaluation of therapy and early detection of relapse. Antibody levels to PGL-I decline rather rapidly after the initiation of chemotherapy[17], suggesting that this glycolipid, abundant in cell-free extracts of infected tissues, is formed by viable bacilli and may be required in rather substantial amounts to sustain a detectable antibody response.

More recently, Brennan has reviewed current knowledge about the biochemical and immunological properties of another carbohydrate-containing component of *M. leprae* membranes, lipoarabinomannan (LAM-B)[17]. In contrast to the reactivity of PGL-I, this highly immunogenic compound shows cross-reactivity with many other mycobacteria and the antibody response which it induces persists for a considerable period after the initiation of chemotherapy. The sensitivity of serological tests based on the use of LAM-B may provide a useful tool for some aspects of epidemiological screening in leprosy control programmes.

Several proteins with specific antigenic determinate, having molecular weights of 12, 18, 28, 36, 65 and 70 kiloDaltons, have been well characterized in *M. leprae*: Draper[18] has characterized the basic cell wall unit.

As mentioned previously, the capacity of *M. leprae* to oxidize D-DOPA (and other related diphenols) has provided the basis for one of the important criteria for its identification. In addition, Wheeler[19] and others have studied a number of metabolic activities, including oxygen metabolism and glycolytic pathways. Extraordinary characteristics, such as deletions in major metabolic pathways, which might explain some of the unique properties of *M. leprae*, have not as yet emerged from these studies, but Wheeler has recently suggested that *M. leprae* does not synthesize its own purines, which may provide a valuable clue to one of the necessary constituents in any proposed artificial medium.

Immunological properties of *M. leprae*

In 1919, Mitsuda demonstrated that lepromatous leprosy patients were unresponsive to heat-treated homogenates of leprosy-infected tissues, while patients with tuberculoid leprosy developed nodular granulomas at the injection sites. The Mitsuda or lepromin reaction has long been used to assess the immunological status of the human host, as will be discussed in another section of this chapter. It also represents a useful criterion for the identification of suspected 'isolates' or infected tissues thought to contain *M. leprae*, since no other mycobacterium shows this characteristic discriminatory pattern of reactivity across the clinical spectrum of leprosy.

The World Health Organization has published guidelines for the preparation of lepromin[20]. *M. leprae* isolated from the tissues of experimentally infected armadillos shows the same immunological characteristics as material from human lesions and is now widely used to prepare skin test antigens. In addition, cell-free extracts prepared from purified armadillo-derived bacilli by rupture in a French pressure cell or by sonication provide useful reageants for evaluating cell-mediated immunity to *M. leprae in vitro* and *in vivo*.

THE PATHOLOGY OF LEPROSY

Introduction

The anatomopathological lesions of leprosy reflect the expression of fundamental factors which intervene in the pathogenesis of the disease. Among these factors, the cell-mediated immune response of the host to the aetiological agent, *M. leprae*, is of particular importance. This response is the determinant factor in the numerous clinical manifestations of leprosy which constitute the clinical spectrum of the disease.

Other factors of importance in the pathology of the disease depend upon particular characteristics of *M. leprae*, including its exceptionally long generation time (11–13 days), low inherent toxicity, and capacity to invade and multiply in peripheral nerves of all sizes, from nerve trunks and bundles to terminal axons in the skin.

The anatomopathological response in leprosy is a chronic granulomatous reaction, except in the lesions of erythema nodosum leprosum (ENL). An acute element is present in ENL reactions, in which immune complexes formed *in situ* between bacillary antigens and antimycobacterial antibodies formed during the course of the infection may play an important role[21]. Cell-mediated reactions of abrupt onset may also occur during upgrading reversal reactions in the intermediate area of the clinical spectrum.

The spectrum of disease is remarkably variable and differences among patients are often very striking, particularly in the intermediate area of the spectrum.

Components of the leprosy granuloma

The principal cellular elements of the chronic granulomatous lesions of leprosy are macrophages in different stages of differentiation and lymphocytes. Polymorphonuclear leukocytes are very rare except in ENL reactional phenomena (Type II reactions).

The study of the granulomatous lesions of leprosy using routine staining of biopsy sections with haematoxylin–eosin often provides a somewhat misleading vision of the cellular components mentioned above. In the tuberculoid pole of the spectrum, both cell types are clearly identified in routine histological preparations. In contrast, the lepromatous granuloma appears to be formed almost exclusively by macrophages, and very few lymphocytes can be identified. The use of monoclonal antibodies which permit the identification of lymphocyte populations and subsets using immunocytochemical techniques provides a more precise vision of the proportion and distribution of lymphocytes in lepromatous granulomas.

Another fundamental component of the leprosy granuloma is, of course, *M. leprae*, in numbers which are directly related to the quality of the cell-mediated immune (CMI) response. Since CMI responses include aspects of both delayed-type hypersensitivity (DTH) and protective immunity, the latter is more clearly related to the numbers of bacilli present in lesions.

The presence of *M. leprae* in leprosy granulomas is a key element not only in the diagnosis of the disease, but in classification within the clinical spectrum, particularly in non-polar, intermediate forms of the disease.

Of the two principal types of cells in leprosy granulomas, macrophages and lymphoid cells, only macrophages show morphological differences in the diverse clinical forms of the disease, with varying degrees of differentiation depending upon the CMI response. Morphological differences are not apparent in the lymphoid cell population using routine staining procedures, but different subpopulations can be readily demonstrated by using appropriate techniques to identify characteristic surface membrane markers. These aspects of the leprosy granuloma will be discussed more fully in the section on immunopathology.

With regard to the macrophages and their modifications throughout the spectrum, the morphological changes are very similar in the early stage of all clinical forms of the disease. These changes appear to correspond to initial macrophage activation observed during the early stages of granuloma formation. The macrophages are elongated, with a fusiform, comma-shaped or indented nucleus. This early stage throughout the spectrum apparently corresponds to the morphological configuration induced by phagocytosis of *M. leprae* and to changes associated with the migration of mononuclear cells into the sites of granuloma formation. The origin of these cells involved in early granuloma formation includes blood monocytes, cells which form the blood vessel endothelium and tissue macrophages which migrate through the cutaneous collagen.

Even at the early stage of granuloma formation, the bacillary component of the incipient lesion provides important information about the eventual position in the clinical spectrum of leprosy that the patient will occupy.

Other aspects of the functional activation of macrophages in leprosy are consequences of the patient's immune response. Appropriate immunological stimuli induce the differentiation of macrophages into epithelioid cells and the formation of Langhans-type giant cells. Epithelioid cells are characterized by a well developed eccentric nucleus with lax chromatin and acidophilic cytoplasm (eosinophilic in routine stains). Their borders with neighbouring cells of the same type are interdigitating and poorly defined. The process of macrophage differentiation toward epithelioid cells shows qualitative differences; incomplete differentiation in the intermediate area of the spectrum may be characterized by epithelioid-type cells containing variable numbers of bacilli in their cytoplasm.

Langhans-type giant cells are probably formed as a result of cellular fusion. They are characterized by acidophilic cytoplasm and multiple nuclei, often arranged in arcs along the periphery of the cell. This type of cell is frequently seen in the tuberculoid pole of the spectrum and in the adjacent borderline tuberculoid region; Langhans giant cells containing bacilli are observed with some frequency in the middle of the spectrum corresponding to borderline leprosy.

Other components of the granuloma such as newly formed blood vessels are abundant in lepromatous granulomas and much less frequent as a shift toward the tuberculoid pole occurs.

Characteristics of the clinical forms of leprosy

Histopathological observations and aspects of the CMI response have been fundamental considerations in different approaches to classification in leprosy. The early Madrid classification (1953) recognized two polar forms of leprosy, lepromatous and tuberculoid disease, as well as a poorly defined intermediate area of borderline or dimorphous leprosy and a separate indeterminate group. Ridley and Jopling[22] were the first authors to propose a more detailed classification of leprosy based on clearly defined histopathological and immunological elements. In this very widely used classification, clear definitions are given for the previously described polar forms of the disease and detailed descriptions of the intermediate area, divided into borderline tuberculoid, borderline and borderline lepromatous forms, are pro-

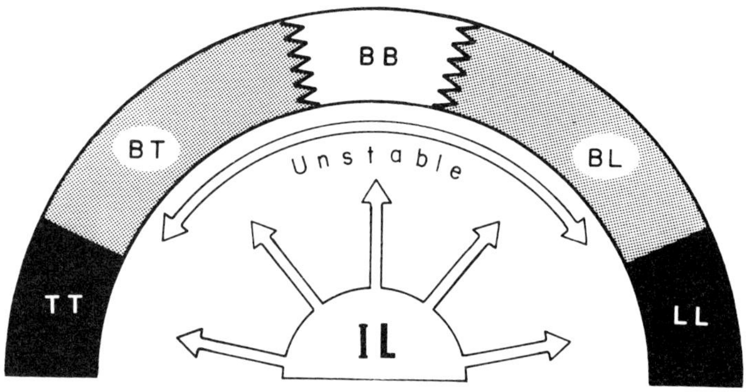

FIGURE 2.3 Clinical-pathological spectrum of leprosy, representing stable polar forms (TT, LL) and unstable intermediate borderline disease (BT, BB, BL). Untreated indeterminate leprosy (IL) may heal spontaneously or progress toward any portion of the spectrum

vided (Figure 2.3). The application of immunological principles and the interpretation of histological expression as a reflection of immunological phenomena have allowed the introduction of a dynamic concept in the spectrum which will be discussed in more detail below.

In order to understand the correlations among diagnosis, clinical lesions, histopathological features, immunological reactivity and bacillary content more clearly, it seems appropriate to examine the Ridley–Jopling classification in some detail. This discussion will be limited to the five most widely recognized groups in the spectrum and to a separate indeterminate group. Only the characteristics of active disease and lesions will be considered, since regressive lesions in the intermediate area often present indeterminate-type characteristics. It should be clear that only well developed lesions provide adequate biopsy specimens for histopathological study.

Polar forms of leprosy

Lepromatous leprosy (LL)

Lepromatous disease is characterized by a long period of incubation and latency. In early stages of the clinical disease, lesions are tenuous, diffuse and erythematous, some showing the colour of a weak iodine solution. These lesions often cover very extensive areas of the body surface and show considerable bilateral symmetry. Particularly in light-skinned patients, the lesions on the extremities often present a reticular aspect which may be confused with livedo reticularis.

As the disease progresses, the skin becomes more infiltrated and

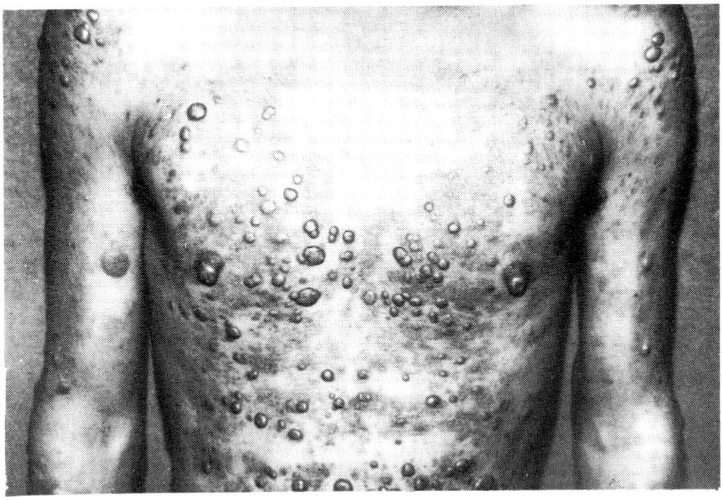

FIGURE 2.4 Polar lepromatous leprosy (LL); multiple nodular lesions distributed symmetrically on the patient's trunk and arms

symmetrical nodules may appear (Figure 2.4). Neurological lesions begin with disturbances in sensitivity; later nerve trunks become enlarged and muscular atrophy with deformities of the hands and feet are observed.

Lepromatous granulomas, when stained by routine methods, are characterized by the presence of undifferentiated macrophages showing variable degrees of vacuolization, from cells containing few small vacuoles to the foamy cells which are typical of LL. Foamy cells are more frequent in lesions of longer evolution and may be almost

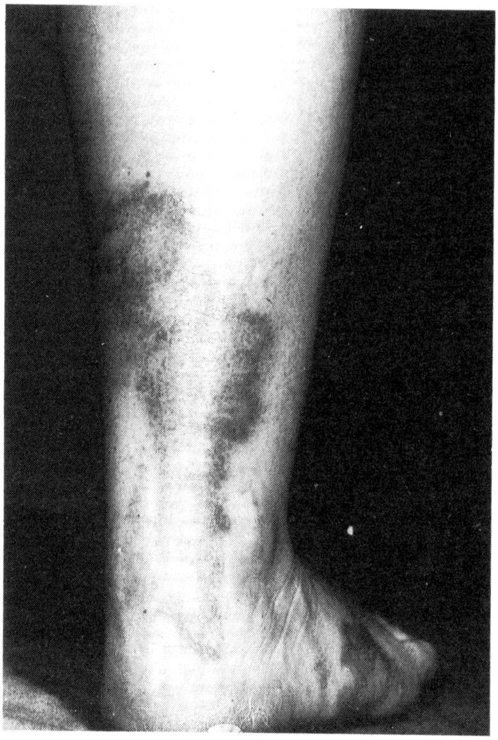

FIGURE 2.8 Borderline tuberculoid (BT) leprosy; few lesions, sharply defined external borders

by moderate systemic manifestations. Histological sections show undifferentiated macrophages as well as macrophages showing varying degrees of epithelioid differentiation and giant cells (Figure 2.10). Large numbers of acid-fast bacilli are observed; lymphocytes, when detectable by routine stains, show a diffuse distribution. We consider it useful to classify all lesions with foci of epithelioid differentiation in the BB group, as well as all patients capable of showing spontaneous upgrading reversal reactions who might otherwise be classified in the borderline lepromatous group; these two phenomena appear to be very closely related. Mitsuda reactivity is not demonstrable in BB patients and lymphocyte transformation tests are very weak or negative.

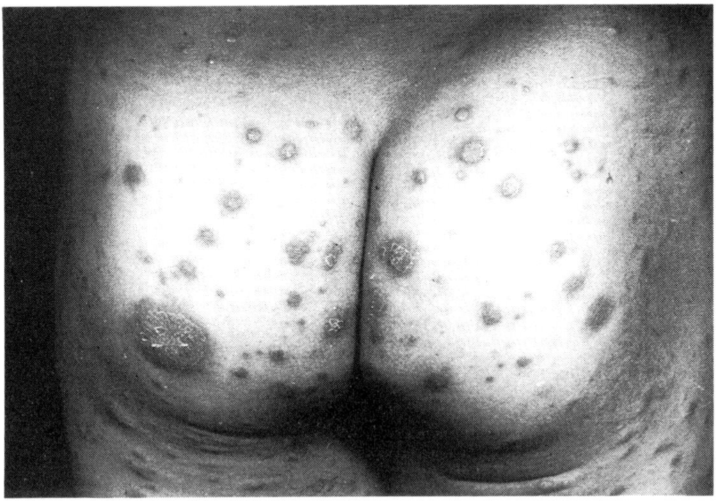

FIGURE 2.9 Borderline (BB) leprosy; numerous lesions with well defined external borders, typical depressed centres

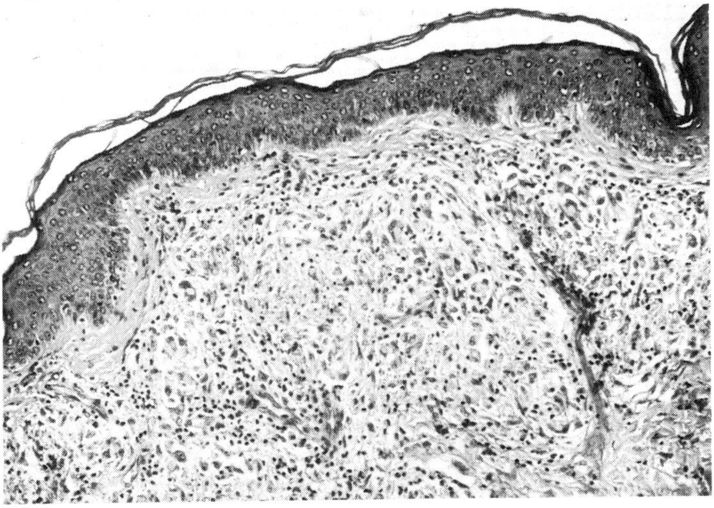

FIGURE 2.10 Histological section of BB. Diffuse infiltration of lymphocytes, macrophages in differing stages of differentiation, without clearly defined structure of an immune granuloma. Original magnification x 160

Borderline lepromatous (BL) leprosy

Borderline lepromatous lesions are very similar to discrete or early forms of polar LL, but the borders of the plaques are more sharply

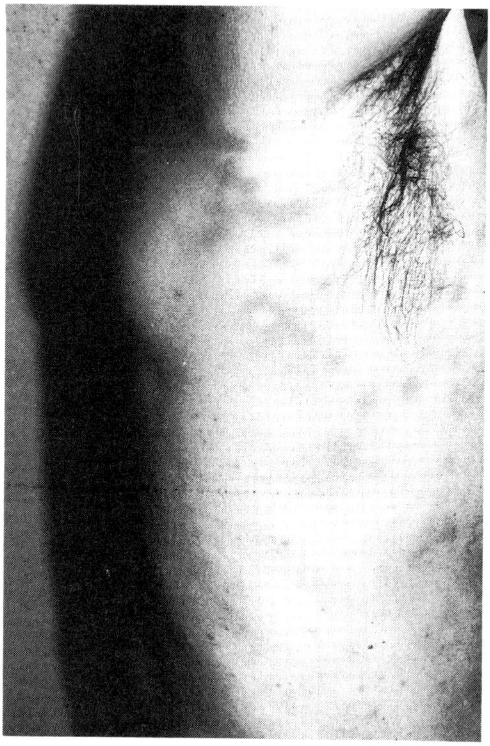

FIGURE 2.11 Borderline lepromatous (BL) leprosy. Numerous plaques with well defined internal borders and diffuse external margins

defined (Figure 2.11). The centre of the lesions often has a normal appearance; the internal border of the infiltration is more sharply defined than the external border, which blends diffusely with the adjacent normal skin. Relapses may be observed in the centre of these lesions. Bilateral symmetry of lesions is not characteristic of BL. Histopathological examination shows a granuloma formed by undifferentiated macrophages, very similar to that observed in early LL. Cellular vacuolization is very limited in BL and very few macrophages with foamy structures are observed; the bacterial population is much smaller than that observed in LL. Patients with BL may show downgrading phenomena with the subsequent development of typical LL lesions. They are always Mitsuda negative.

It should be emphasized that all intermediate forms of leprosy are relatively unstable and their position in the clinical spectrum may shift during disease evolution. This is particularly true of BB leprosy, which is infrequently diagnosed in most parts of the world. This characteristic is in marked contrast with the stability of polar forms of the disease.

Indeterminate leprosy

This form of leprosy should be clearly distinguished from self-healing lesions. The latter possess a non-progressive character and do not represent well defined clinical forms of leprosy; they appear to be the expression of self-healing, limited infection.

The clinical lesions of indeterminate leprosy consist of a single or few hypopigmented patches which show anaesthesia (Figure 2.12). Depending upon the immunological capacity of the patient, these initial hypopigmented lesions may progress toward any of the well defined forms of the clinical spectrum, showing either upgrading or downgrading reactivity. The hypopigmented lesions of indeterminate leprosy must be distinguished from the secondary hypopigmented residual lesions observed during the involution of BB and BL; the latter are much more numerous and histopathological examination reveals a larger bacterial population in the interior of nerves.

The histological structure of the indeterminate lesion is characterized by moderate lympho-histiocytic infiltration of blood vessels and especially of cutaneous nerves. Isolated acid-fast bacilli may be found within nerves (Figure 2.13) and in pilo-erector muscles. Clearly, this type of discrete inflammatory reaction is non-specific, and only the presence of isolated bacilli provides the criterion necessary for definitive diagnosis.

The immunological reactivity of patients with indeterminate leprosy is variable; they may be Mitsuda positive or show persisting Mitsuda negativity. The latter group is associated with poor prognosis and requires more aggressive therapy.

While we have emphasized the pathology of cutaneous lesions in this discussion, the granulomas of LL and intermediate borderline

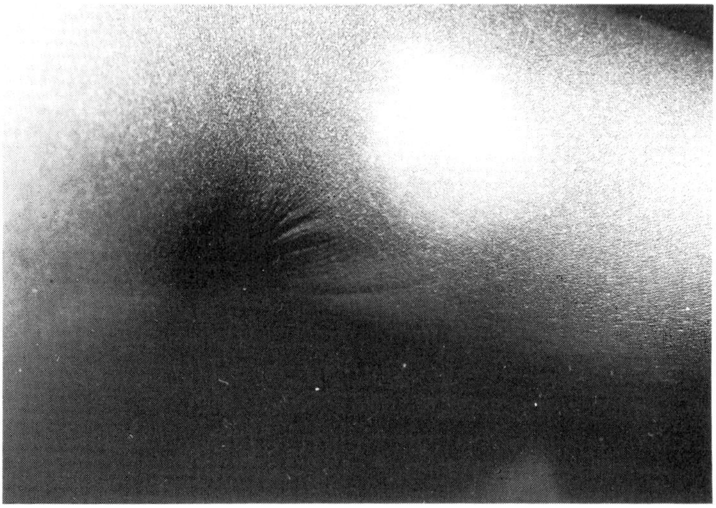

FIGURE 2.12 Characteristic hypopigmented macule of indeterminate leprosy

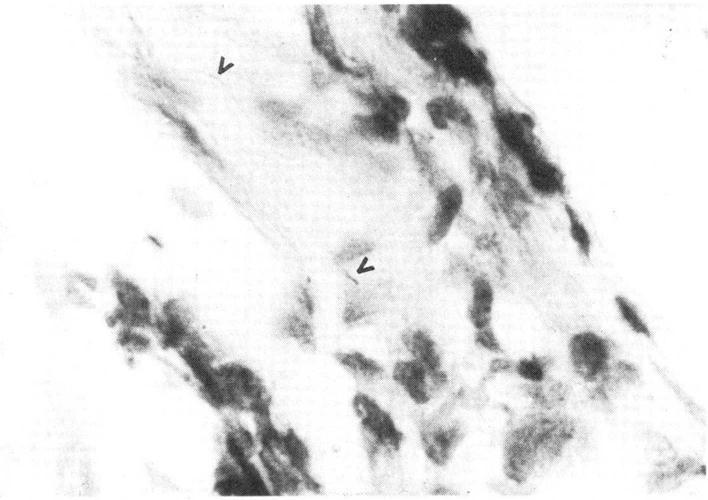

FIGURE 2.13 Acid-fast bacilli, indicated by arrows, within a superficial nerve in indeterminate leprosy

groups are often localized in nerve trunks and viscera, with the exception of the lungs, brain and digestive tract. The ocular lesions of leprosy represent one of the most serious causes of disability, and specialized references should be consulted by interested readers[23].

IMMUNOLOGICAL ASPECTS OF LEPROSY

Introduction

The varying pathological manifestations of leprosy described in the previous section of this chapter depend upon a complex host–parasite relationship in which the host's capacity to develop a competent immunological response plays a fundamental role. The unique capacity of *M. leprae* to invade peripheral nerves as well as phagocytic and endothelial cells of many organs and its predilection for cooler tissues of the body are largely responsible for the distribution of lesions in the human infection. For many years, prolonged and intimate contact with infected individuals was considered to be a requisite for transmission. More recent immunological and epidemiological evidence clearly suggests that *M. leprae* may, in fact, be quite highly contagious, but that most individuals develop a strong protective immune response and the infection is controlled during one or repeated subclinical episodes. While the pathogenic characteristics of *M. leprae* mentioned above cannot be overlooked, leprosy is frequently considered to be an immunological as well as infectious disease, since so many of its features are best described in terms of the host's immune response.

The enormous complexity of the immune system cannot be adequately dealt with in this rather brief communication, but some knowledge of its role in leprosy is indispensable in understanding the disease more clearly. For didactic purposes, it remains useful to consider two broad categories of immune responsiveness: humoral immunity, mediated by antibodies or immunoglobulins, and cell-mediated immunity, mediated by thymus-dependent (T) lymphocytes. These two types of reactivity are intimately interrelated in their development, expression and regulation; each is characterized by the development of protective, beneficial reactions for the host and by hypersensitivity reactions resulting in damage to host tissues. In addition to the large number of cells and soluble mediators recognized as integral components of the immune system (Figure 2.14), recent evidence suggests important interaction with neurological and endocrine systems. The genetic basis of many aspects of immunological responsiveness has been very clearly established, and the influence of environmental factors has not yet been adequately assessed in many

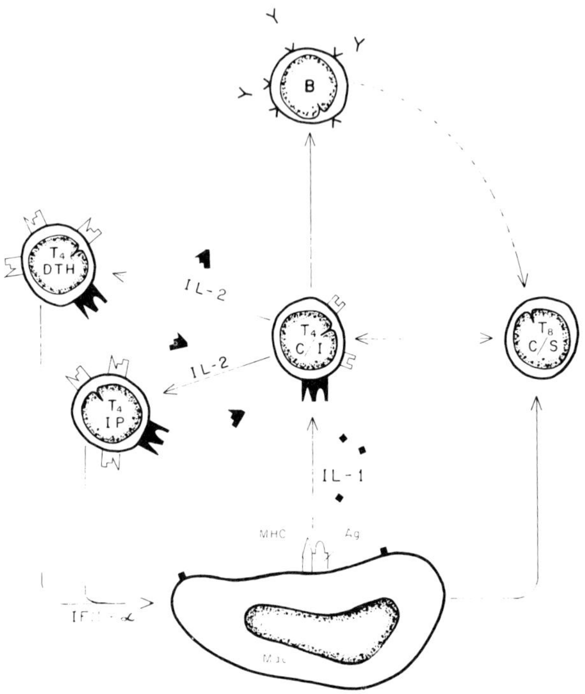

FIGURE 2.14 Principal cells and soluble mediators involved in the immune response. Cells include macrophages (Mac), T lymphocytes (T_4) cooperator/inducer cells; subsets responsible for delayed-type hypersensitivity (DTH) and protective immunity (IP); T_8 cytotoxic/suppressor cells) and B lymphocytes (antibody producer precursors). Soluble mediators include interleukins (IL-1 and IL-2) and gamma interferon (IFN-γ). MHC = molecules associated with the major histocompatibility complex; Ag = antigen

human infections. In this section, an effort will be made to summarize the more relevant aspects of this extraordinarily complex situation in leprosy.

The antibody response in leprosy

M. leprae is an obligate intracellular pathogen; protective immunity depends predominantly, if not exclusively, upon T lymphocyte, cell-mediated immunity. Nevertheless, the micro-organism stimulates specific and non-specific antibody responses which play a role in some aspects of the pathology of leprosy, and the antibody response may offer tools for immuno-epidemiological studies, detection of sub-clinical infection and monitoring clinical disease.

M. leprae is characterized by a highly complex antigenic structure, containing numerous components in its wall, membranes and protoplasm which stimulate the synthesis of circulating antibodies. Many of the immunogenic components of *M. leprae* are shared with other mycobacteria and related micro-organisms; others, such as the phenolic glycolipid (PGL-I) referred to previously, elicit a highly specific antibody response. Specific antigenic determinants or epitopes have been identified on at least six proteins of *M. leprae*, having molecular weights of 12, 18, 28, 37, 65 and 70 kiloDaltons, using monoclonal antibodies derived from hybridomas produced by the fusion of myeloma cells with single antibody-producing cells.

There is no evidence that the numerous antimycobacterial antibodies produced in response to infection by *M. leprae* play any direct role in protective immunity. Specific and non-specific antimycobacterial antibodies occur with the greatest frequency and highest titres precisely in the most severe, progressive forms of the disease, toward the lepromatous pole of the clinical spectrum. No antibodies of a particular specificity have as yet been associated with any clinical form of leprosy; antibody titres in general appear to be closely related to the bacterial load present in the patient's tissues.

While antimycobacterial antibodies have not been associated with protective mechanisms in leprosy, they have been implicated in some of the pathological manifestations of lepromatous disease, including erythema nosodum leprosum and immune-complex glomerulonephritis, as discussed in the following section.

The concept that patients suffering from lepromatous leprosy are immunologically 'anergic' or non-reactive must be re-examined in terms of this immunologically fascinating dissociation which they show between synthesis of antimycobacterial antibodies and development of CMI reactivity to *M. leprae*. Tools such as the hybridoma technique for producing monoclonal antibodies and procedures for isolating T-cell clones may provide answers to some of the most provocative questions in leprosy research. Are the same antigenic determinants responsible for stimulating antibody (B cell) and T-cell responses? Are there specific epitopes associated with protective responses? With so many common features in the induction of T- and B-cell responses, what immunoregulatory pathways permit the expression of one of these responses (antibody synthesis) and the absence of protective and hypersensitivity expressions of CMI?

In spite of their apparent lack of importance in protective immunity in leprosy, studies of the antibody response to *M. leprae* bear an extraordinary potential in at least five areas of study:

(1) Immunoepidemiological studies, based on the use of specific natural or synthetic antigens to detect infection rates and distribution.

(2) Development of sensitive tests to detect subclinical infection. Tests for the detection of antibodies to PGL-I, though relatively insensitive, provide a first step in this area of study.

(3) Monitoring of the efficacy of therapy. Antibodies to PGL-I, mostly of the IgM class, decline rather rapidly after the initiation of chemotherapy and would appear to reflect numbers of viable bacilli in the tissues.

(4) Early detection of relapse, drug resistance or re-infection. Rising titres of antibodies during the course of therapy or after its suspension against almost any antigenic preparation of *M. leprae* would provide useful information in this area of study.

(5) Evaluation of immunoprophylactic preparations and protocols. If epitopes which stimulate protective responses can be identified, and if they stimulate both CMI and antibody responses, the latter may be much easier to evaluate in large populations. Following the same line of thought, the stimulation of antibodies to so-called 'suppressor epitopes' might provide one criterion for screening out less promising vaccination protocols.

The prerequisites for useful serological tests at the field level include high specificity for *M. leprae*, high sensitivity for the detection of weak antibody responses, and the use of relatively straightforward tests which do not require enormous technological support or unstable or costly reagents. At present, no universal test is available which fulfils all of the criteria outlined above. Enzyme-linked immunoassays (ELISA tests) have become popular in developing countries, since they are highly sensitive, give quantitative data, and make use of stable reagents. PGL-I possesses the degree of specificity required for these tests, but is of limited sensitivity; soluble extracts of *M. leprae* and antigenic preparations such as the membrane-associated lipoarabinomannan, LAM-B, are more sensitive but show extensive cross-reactivity with other mycobacteria and related micro-organisms.

The molecular biology of *M. leprae* has been characterized by spectacular advances in knowledge in the last decade, due in large part to the active research programme developed by the IMMLEP programme of the World Health Organization. One of the great challenges not fully confronted in these studies has been evaluation of possible practical applications of these advances in appropriate field studies. A notable exception is represented in the use of native PGL-I and of neoglycoproteins containing the same carbohydrate determinants in many field studies, for which Dr Patrick Brennan deserves due recognition.

In concluding this discussion of the antibody response in leprosy, it should be noted that many patients suffering from multibacillary leprosy produce low levels of autoantibodies to their own tissues. To our knowledge, there is little evidence that these antibodies contribute to the pathology of the disease or that they produce autoimmune pathology. At least two mechanisms, not mutually exclusive, might be invoked to explain the formation of these antibodies: neoantigens may be formed at the sites of chronic inflammatory lesions, which would stimulate the production of self-reacting antibodies, and *M. leprae*, which shares the adjuvant activity characteristic of other mycobacteria, may facilitate the development of an immune response to native host antigens.

Cell-mediated immunity in leprosy

The clinical, histopathological and immunological spectrum of leprosy (Figure 2.15) depends upon the capacity of the infected host to develop a competent cell-mediated immune response to *M. leprae*, and all of the clinical forms of the disease probably reflect varying degrees of immunological abnormality. As in many other infections produced by

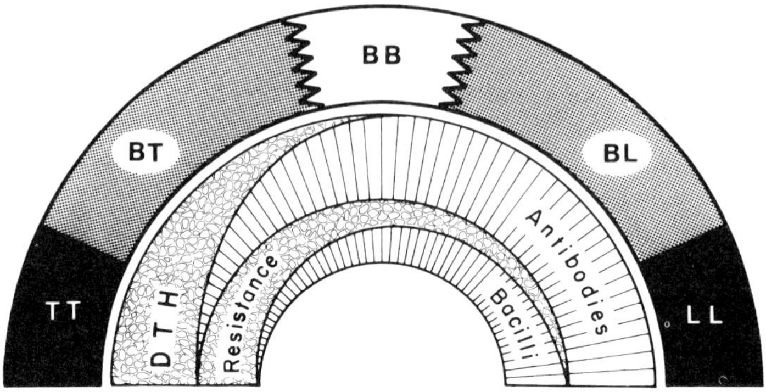

FIGURE 2.15 Clinical immunological spectrum of leprosy. Delayed-type hypersensitivity (DTH) and resistance decline throughout the spectrum with the shift from TT toward LL. This same shift is accompanied by an increase in antimycobacterial antibodies and bacilli in lesions

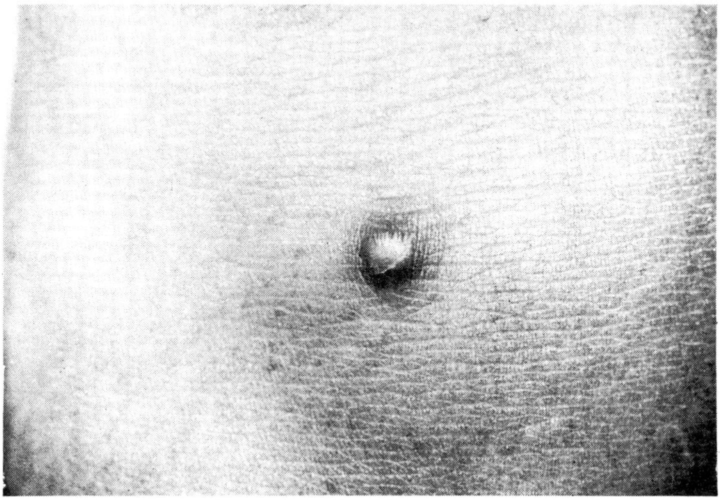

FIGURE 2.16 Positive Mitsuda reaction, 21 days after the intradermal injection of 16×10^6 heat-killed *M. leprae* in a patient with tuberculoid leprosy

obligate intracellular micro-organisms, development of a protective immune response occurs when specifically sensitized T lymphocytes activate the macrophages or other host cells harboring the infective agent, resulting in death of the micro-organism. Macrophage activation is not due to direct interaction with T cells, but occurs in response to the synthesis of soluble mediators, of which gamma interferon (IFN-γ) appears to be the most important. T cells which bear the CD4 membrane antigen appear to be the principal sources of IFN-γ production. Another mechanism for destroying infected cells is cytolysis or cytotoxicity, mediated by a T-cell subpopulation bearing the CD8 membrane marker or by 'killer' cells. The first mechanism involving macrophage activation has received much more attention as the most important mechanism involved in the protective response to *M. leprae*.

Development of T-cell protective immunity is usually accompanied during the course of natural infections by the development of delayed-type hypersensitivity (DTH) to the same micro-organism, and leprosy is no exception to this generalization. Most, if not all, of the *in vivo* and *in vitro* tests designed to measure CMI in reality measure different aspects of DTH, and must be interpreted with some caution in terms of the relationship between positive tests and protective immunity.

The most widely used procedures for evaluating CMI in leprosy are skin tests and lymphocyte transformation tests. The value of the information provided by skin tests is often underestimated; the judicious use of such tests in epidemiological surveys, prognosis of early indeterminate leprosy, evaluation of the immunological status of healthy contacts, detection of high-risk populations, and evaluation of immunotherapeutic and immunoprophylactic procedures allows the study of large populations far beyond the capacity of most centres which carry out *in vitro* tests.

Since its description by Mitsuda in 1919, most skin testing in leprosy has been based on the use of heat-killed preparations of *M. leprae* from human tissue or, more recently, of armadillo-derived bacilli. These 'integral lepromins' induce immune granulomatous reactions (Figure 2.16) which are usually read after 21–30 days, and reflect the capacity of the host to develop a CMI reaction to *M. leprae*, whether he has been exposed to or infected by *M. leprae* or not. Positive reactivity in the lepromin test has often been interpreted as a correlate of protective immunity, but the immune granulomatous reaction is probably in reality an *in vivo* manifestation of DTH.

Early studies of Fernandez noted the presence of a classical tuberculin-type DTH reaction at 48–72 hours in many patients injected with lepromin. This early reactivity is attributed to soluble antigen present in the lepromin preparations. In recent years, several types of soluble extracts have been used for the evaluation of CMI in leprosy patients and healthy individuals; these preparations include soluble extracts prepared from purified armadillo-derived *M. leprae* by rupture under pressure[24] or sonication[25] and subsequent removal of insoluble debris by centrifugation. Tests with soluble preparations measure pre-existing hypersensitivity. In Venezuela, reactions with soluble antigens have been widely used to assess the response of leprosy patients to immunotherapy, and to evaluate subsequent reactivity to immunoprophylactic stimulation with a mixture of heat-killed *M. leprae* and BCG. In another application of considerable interest, skin tests are used as one criterion to identify healthy individuals at high risk, in conjunction with epidemiological studies[26]. This application is based on the identification of both household and non-household contacts of leprosy patients through epidemiological screening; contacts capable of developing a competent immune response to *M. leprae* would be expected to give positive skin tests due to their often prolonged exposure to the micro-organism. Those contacts who give negative tests are considered to be at high risk to develop multibacillary leprosy and are candidates for immunoprophylaxis. The presence of antibodies to PGL-I in these negative reactors is strong presumptive evidence of subclinical multibacillary infection. This interpretation of skin-test reactivity in terms of risk places an unusually strong emphasis on the significance of negative responses.

All skin test reagents in use at present are extraordinarily complex mixtures of antigens, some of which are specific for *M. leprae* and others which are shared with many other related micro-organisms. Therefore, positive reactions cannot be ascribed to infection with *M. leprae* and these preparations are not useful in studying infection rates. The same limitation exists in *in vitro* tests such as the lymphocyte transformation test, leukocyte migration inhibition tests and others. Bearing this limitation in mind, all tests which measure CMI to *M. leprae*-derived antigens show relatively high levels of activity at the tuberculoid or resistant pole of the clinical spectrum; this reactivity decreases across the spectrum and becomes negative in borderline lepromatous and lepromatous patients[27]. CMI reactivity is related inversely to the presence of circulating antimycobacterial antibodies.

The absence of CMI to *M. leprae* in lepromatous disease is a highly specific phenomenon, though advanced disease may be associated with some degree of non-specific immunodepression. There is considerable clinical as well as experimental evidence supporting this observation; patients with lepromatous leprosy do not show unusual susceptibility to other infections or illnesses associated with depressed CMI, such as viral or mycotic infections or tumours. The incapacity to develop CMI to *M. leprae* clearly exists in some individuals before they develop clinical disease, and persistent Mitsuda negativity in healthy individuals may be an important factor in the subsequent development of lepromatous disease in exposed individuals[28]. The basis for this lack of reactivity in apparently healthy individuals remains unclear. Several possibilities exist: specific CMI may be actively suppressed in very early subclinical stages of infection; route or intensity of exposure, nutritional status, intercurrent infections, previous exposure to other mycobacteria and genetic factors may all contribute to varying degrees in the subsequent development of a competent response.

It is generally accepted that most lepromatous patients neither develop nor recover CMI to *M. leprae* after successful chemotherapy, and that they remain susceptible to re-infection or to relapse from dormant micro-organisms or 'persisters' for the remainder of their lives. Nevertheless, studies in our Institute have demonstrated that CMI to *M. leprae* can be induced in 65–75% of lepromatous patients by adequate immunotherapy with repeated injections of a mixture of viable BCG and heat-killed *M. leprae*[26,29], indicating that non-reactivity is not an irreversible condition in many patients. Induction of CMI is achieved much more readily in patients with early Mitsuda-negative leprosy. These observations, together with the immuno-epidemiological approach to the identification of healthy individuals at high risk described above and the observation of skin-test conversion in healthy contacts after a single injection of the *M. leprae*–BCG mixture, form the basis for our approach to the immunoprophylaxis of leprosy.

An enormous effort has been devoted to try to identify the antigen-specific defect responsible for the development of lepromatous leprosy, and presumably to a lesser degree throughout the clinical spectrum of the disease. Some of the factors implicated are summarized in the following section on the immunopathology of the disease. Perhaps special mention should be made here of the possible role of T-suppressor cells. There is considerable evidence that a competent CMI response depends upon an adequate balance of T-helper (T4) and T-suppressor (T8) cells. Perhaps this relationship has been most thoroughly studied in experimental leishmaniasis, a parasitic disease which shares many of the immunological features of leprosy. Mehra, Bloom and collaborators have presented strong arguments for the importance of an active T-cell suppressor response in lepromatous leprosy[30]; PGL-I and neoglycoconjugates bearing the same carbohydrates have been shown by this group to elicit suppressor activity[31]. Nevertheless, failure to confirm these observations in other laboratories and other observations such as the non-specific suppressor activity of various *M. leprae* components, including LAM-B[32], suggest that active suppressor mechanisms must be interpreted with some restraint, in spite of their evident intellectual appeal.

The development of specific antigenic preparations for the evaluation of CMI in leprosy remains as one of the great challenges in the field, and almost surely will require the ingenious application of genetic engineering, T-cell cloning and other techniques of biotechnology. At present it seems fair to say that we have no knowledge about the nature of the antigenic determinants which induce protective immunity to *M. leprae*, nor their relationship to determinants which induce DTH, cell-mediated cytotoxicity, suppression or antibody synthesis. It has been proposed that a 'suppressor determinant', such as PGL-I, could shut down the CMI response to all of the common and specific antigens of *M. leprae*, but the patients with this defect develop reactivity to the specific antigens of other mycobacteria, such as BCG, which share many of the same common antigens. This reflects a discriminatory immunological response almost beyond comprehension in terms of our present knowledge. There is no evidence yet which would suggest an equally powerful 'protective determinant'; indeed an effective protective response may require activity to multiple determinants, some of them specific and others non-specific. All of these questions provide an extraordinary stimulus for the continued interest in the immunological aspects of leprosy.

THE IMMUNOPATHOLOGY OF LEPROSY

Introduction

To review briefly what has been said in previous sections, *Mycobacterium leprae* is a micro-organism which is remarkably devoid of inherent characteristics associated with pathogenicity. No exotoxins or endotoxins with pathogenic consequences for the host have been described. Infected tissues in lepromatous leprosy may contain many millions of bacilli per gram of tissue, with clinical manifestations sometimes limited to relatively discrete tissue infiltration, imperceptible to the untrained eye. The principal characteristics of *M. leprae* which produce the most serious consequences in leprosy include its capacity to invade and multiply within Schwann cells and other structures of peripheral nerves, and to multiply in histiocytes, endothelial cells and other cell types in many organs of the body. Apart from these characteristics, the immunopathology of leprosy can be described almost exclusively in terms of the consequences of the host's immune response to *M. leprae*. Both cell-mediated and immune complex pathology may be involved in lesions of skin, nerves, bones, joints, eyes and kidneys.

Most infections caused by *M. leprae* are probably healed by an effective immune response during one or repeated subclinical episodes. Studies using a soluble extract of *M. leprae* in Venezuela have shown that about 75% of the contacts living in highly endemic areas have developed an immune response to specific or common antigens of *M. leprae* with no clinical manifestations of disease[26]. Health workers become sensitized to *M. leprae* after relatively brief contact with patients suffering from leprosy. There is considerable evidence of this type which suggests that all clinical manifestations of leprosy may represent some degree of immunological deficiency in the affected host. It has been widely accepted for many years that this deficiency is highly antigen-specific and that its pathological effects are largely limited to the activities of some T lymphocyte subpopulations.

Tuberculoid leprosy

Tuberculoid leprosy is accompanied by many of the manifestations of a competent cell-mediated immune response to *M. leprae*. Lesions are few; mycobacteria are often detected only with difficulty. *In vivo* and *in vitro* manifestations of cell-mediated immunity (CMI) to specific and common antigens of *M. leprae* can be demonstrated by tests for delayed-type hypersensitivity (DTH) *in vivo*, including 48-hour skin tests with soluble extract of *M. leprae* and Mitsuda-type reactions. *In vitro* counterparts of DTH, including lymphoblastic transformation and synthesis of lymphokines, are positive in tests employing diverse preparations of *M. leprae*. Conventional histopathology demonstrates an immune granuloma formed principally by lymphocytes and differentiated macrophages, including epithelioid cells and Langhans giant cells. More recent immunocytology utilizing monoclonal antibodies reveals a relatively high (>1) $CD4^+/CD8^+$ ratio of T cells, large numbers of cells producing interleukin-2 (IL-2) and bearing IL-2 receptors, and localization of T cells bearing the $CD8^+$ marker largely limited to the peripheral lymphocytic mantle[33,34] (Figure 2.17). Hyperplasia of Langerhans cells is observed in the dermis and epidermis of these lesions. Epidermal keratinocytes are HLA-DR^+, probably reflecting stimulation by gamma interferon (IFN-γ)[35]. In spite of this abundant evidence of T-cell reactivity in tuberculoid leprosy, protective immunity in these patients is incomplete and they usually require chemotherapy to resolve their infections.

Nerve damage in tuberculoid leprosy

Undoubtedly the most serious consequence of the inability to eliminate *M. leprae* in patients with tuberculoid leprosy is manifest in severe damage to peripheral nerves. The precise mechanisms of this damage are not clear, but two factors of undoubted importance have been recognized, both reflecting the consequence of the host's immune response to the presence of *M. leprae* in nerves. First, a profuse mononuclear infiltrate may be produced when mycobacterial antigens react with sensitized T cells and the latter liberate factors which recruit non-sensitized cells. Second, the biologically active products of this

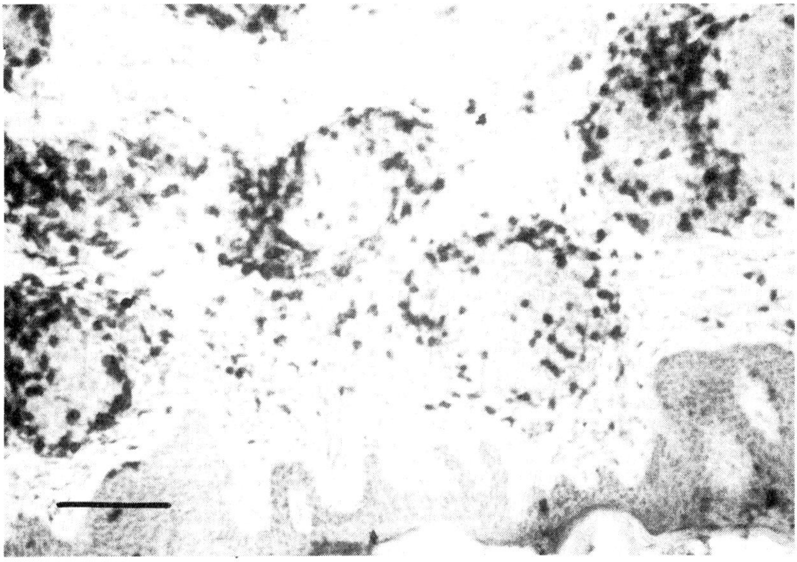

FIGURE 2.17 Immunoperoxidase staining of T $CD8^{+}$ lymphocytes (cytotoxic/suppressor cells) in a tuberculoid leprosy granuloma, showing characteristic distribution in the peripheral mantle. Bar = 40 μm. Photo courtesy Dr F. J. Tapia

infiltrate, including diverse cytotoxic lymphokines and monokines, lysosomal enzymes, etc. may contribute substantially to the mechanical disorganization and dysfunction caused by an abundant infiltrate within a sheathed nerve; these biological mediators may be of even greater importance in damaging fine nerve endings and filaments. Cytolysis of Schwann cells harboring *M. leprae* may contribute to nerve damage. An element of autoimmunity has been postulated as a contributing factor in nerve damage in tuberculoid leprosy, based on the formation of neoantigens within the inflammatory lesion and adjuvant effects of even a limited number of mycobacteria. Neural autoantibodies have been described in leprosy by Wright *et al.*[36]. There is no satisfactory model for the peripheral nerve damage caused by *M. leprae* at present, although some of the demyelinating diseases share common features. Infection of adult trigeminal neurons from the rabbit with *M. leprae* may provide a useful model for studying some aspects of nerve damage.

Borderline leprosy

The intermediate borderline forms of leprosy represent an extremely varied immunopathological group. These clinical manifestations may be more frequent than polar forms of disease in many populations. They are frequently unstable; both upgrading reactions reflecting an increase in CMI and downgrading reactions reflecting a shift toward less resistant forms of the disease are observed.

Reactions in borderline leprosy

The abrupt changes in cellular immunity which occur during upgrading episodes in borderline leprosy are often accompanied by reversal reactions (Type 1 reactions) which affect both skin and nerves. Skin reversal reactions are characterized by erythema, oedema and tenderness, usually within previously existing lesions[37,38].

The dramatic onset of neurological manifestations may require the use of relatively high doses of corticosteroids or, in some circumstances, surgical decompression, in order to prevent permanent damage. The mechanisms of nerve damage in upgrading reversal reactions are similar to those described above in tuberculoid leprosy. The abrupt onset may reflect a considerably larger bacillary population in the nerves in borderline leprosy, accompanied by a significant change in the activity of lymphocyte subpopulations (i.e. an increase in the proportion of DTH effector cells in relation to suppressor cells).

Nielsen *et al.*[39] have analysed the phenotypic characteristics of cellular infiltrates in leprosy neuritis. Interestingly enough, this study confirms others demonstrating that classification based on skin and nerve biopsies often shows important discrepancies. While lymphocytic infiltrates in nerves were more diffuse than those in cutaneous granulomatous lesions, $CD4^+/CD8^+$ ratios and cells bearing IL-2 receptors (TAC^+) were generally high in paucibacillary nerve biopsies; both values decreased in multibacillary nerve lesions.

Lepromatous leprosy

Lepromatous leprosy (LL) is characterized by multiple lesions which may cover essentially the entire body surface, huge numbers of bacilli, and negative responses in the immunological tests which measure DTH to antigens of *M. leprae in vivo* and *in vitro*. There is considerable evidence that patients suffering from LL do not constitute a homogeneous group. The capacity of lymphocytes from some LL patients to respond to *M. leprae* in the presence of exogenous IL-2[40] may reflect the presence of a group of relative 'responders' among LL patients. Atypical, paucibacillary LL has been described. Our own experience in the immunotherapy of lepromatous patients suggests the presence of a subspectrum within the LL group[24,26,41]. Perhaps 25–35% of these patients do not respond after ten or more bimonthly treatments with *M. leprae* and BCG, based on clinical and histopathological criteria; the others respond after variable numbers of treatments. Some appear

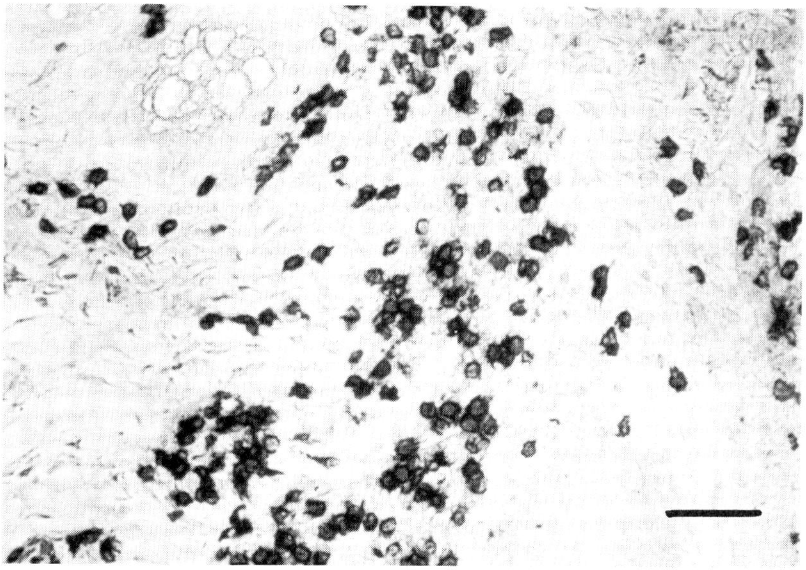

FIGURE 2.18 Cytotoxic/suppressor T CD8$^+$ cells in a lepromatous lesion, revealed by immunoperoxidase staining. Note disperse distribution throughout the granuloma. Bar = 20 μm. Photo courtesy Dr F. J. Tapia

Mycobacterium leprae from other mycobacteria through routine staining techniques. *Int. J. Lepr.*, **40,** 130–2

7. Prabhakaran, K. and Kirchheimer, W. F. (1966). Use of 3,4-dihydroxyphenylalanine oxidation in the identification of *Mycobacterium leprae*. *J. Bacteriol.*, **92,** 1267–8
8. Rees, R. J. W. (1985). The microbiology of leprosy. In Hastings, R. C. (ed.) *Leprosy*. pp. 31–52. (Edinburgh: Churchill Livingstone)
9. Ridley, D. S. (1958). Therapeutic trials in leprosy using serial biopsies. *Lepr. Rev.*, **29,** 45–52
10. Rees, R. J. W. and Valentine, R. C. (1962). The appearance of dead leprosy bacilli by light and electron microscopy. *Int. J. Lepr.*, **30,** 1–9
11. McRae, D. H. and Shepard, C. C. (1971). Relationship between the staining quality of *Mycobacterium leprae* and infectivity for mice. *Infect. Immun.*, **3,** 116–20
12. Shepard, C. C. and McRae, D. H. (1965). *Mycobacterium leprae* in mice: minimal infectious dose, relationship between staining quality and infectivity and effect of cortisone. *J. Bacteriol.*, **89,** 365–72
13. Rees, R. J. W. (1971). The impact of experimental human leprosy in the mouse on leprosy research. *Int. J. Lepr.*, **39,** 201–15
14. Shepard, C. C. and McRae, D. H. (1971). Hereditary characteristic that varies among isolates of *Mycobacterium leprae*. *Infect. Immun.*, **3,** 121–6
15. Walsh, G. P., Storrs, E. E., Meyers, W. M. and Binford, C. H. (1977). Naturally acquired leprosy-like disease in the nine-banded armadillo (*Dasypus novemcinctus*). Recent epizootiologic findings. *J. Reticuloendothel. Soc.*, **22,** 363–8
16. Brennan, P. J. and Barrow, W. W. (1980). Evidence for species-specific lipid antigens in *Mycobacterium leprae*. *Int. J. Lepr.*, **48,** 382–7
17. Brennan, P. J. (1986). The carbohydrate-containing antigens of *Mycobacterium leprae*. *Lepr. Rev., Suppl. 2*, **57,** 39–51
18. Draper, P. (1984). Wall biosynthesis: a possible site of action for new antimycobacterial drugs. *Int. J. Lepr.*, **52,** 527–32
19. Wheeler, P. R. (1986). Enzymes and other biochemically active components of mycobacteria. *Lepr. Rev.*, **57,** *Suppl. 2*, 21–32
20. World Health Organization Memorandum (1979). Recommended safety requirements for the preparation of lepromin. *Bull. WHO*, **57,** 921–3
21. Wemambu, S. N. C., Turk, J. L., Waters, M. F. R. and Rees, R. J. W. (1969). ENL – a clinical manifestation of the Arthus phenomenon. *Lancet*, **2,** 933–5
22. Ridley, D. S. and Jopling, W. C. (1966). Classification of leprosy according to immunity: a five-group system. *Int. J. Lepr.*, **34,** 255–73
23. Brand, M. E. and Ffytche, T. J. (1985). Eye complications of leprosy. In Hastings, R. C. (ed.) *Leprosy*. pp. 223–42. (Edinburgh: Churchill Livingstone)
24. Convit, J., Aranzazu, N., Ulrich, M., Pinardi, M. E., Reyes, O. and Alvarado, J. (1982). Immunotherapy with a mixture of *Mycobacterium leprae* and BCG in different forms of leprosy and in Mitsuda-negative contacts. *Int. J. Lepr.*, **50,** 415–24
25. Shield, M. J., Stanford, J. L., Garbajosa, G., Draper, P. and Rees, R. J. W. (1982). The epidemiological evaluation, in Burma, of the skin test reagent LRA6; a cell-free extract from armadillo-derived *Mycobacterium leprae*. 1. Leprosy patients. *Int. J. Lepr.*, **50,** 436–45
26. Convit, J., Aranzazu, N., Zuñiga, M., Ulrich, M., Pinardi, M. E., Castellazzi, Z.

and Alvarado, J. (1983). Immunotherapy and immunoprophylaxis of leprosy. *Lepr. Rev.*, Special Issue, 47–60
27. Myrvang, B., Godal, T., Ridley, D.S., Froland, S.S. and Song, Y.K. (1973). Immune responsiveness to *Mycobacterium leprae* and other mycobacterial antigens throughout the clinical and histopathological spectrum of leprosy. *Clin. Exp. Immunol.*, **14,** 541–53
28. Dharmendra and Chatterjee, K.R. (1955). Prognostic value of the lepromin test in contacts of leprosy cases. *Lepr. India*, **27,** 149
29. Convit, J., Aranzazu, N., Ulrich, M., Pinardi, M.E., Castellanos, P.L. and Zuñiga, M. (1986). Vaccination in leprosy. In Casal, M. (ed.) *Mycobacteria of Clinical Interest*. pp. 336–44. (Amsterdam: Elsevier Science Publishers BV)
30. Mehra, V., Mason, L.H., Fields, J.P. and Bloom, B. (1979). Lepromin-induced suppressor cells in patients with leprosy. *J. Immunol.*, **123,** 1813–17
31. Mehra, V., Brennan, P.J., Rada, E., Convit, J. and Bloom, B.R. (1984). Lymphocyte suppression in leprosy induced by unique *M. leprae* glycolipid. *Nature (London)*, **308,** 194–6
32. Kaplan, G., Gandhi, R.R., Weinstein, D.E., Levis, W.R., Patarroyo, M.E., Brennan, P.J. and Cohn, Z.A. (1987). *Mycobacterium leprae* antigen-induced suppression of T cell proliferation *in vitro*. *J. Immunol.*, **138,** 3028–34
33. Van Voorhis, W.C., Kaplan, G., Sarno, E.N., Horwitz, M.A., Steinman, R.M., Levis, W.R., Nogueira, N., Hair, L.S., Gatass, C.R., Arrick, B.A. and Cohn, Z.A. (1982). The cutaneous infiltrates of leprosy, cellular characteristics and the predominant T-cell phenotypes. *N. Engl. J. Med.*, **307,** 1593–7
34. Modlin, R.L., Hofman, F.M., Horwitz, D.A., Husmann, L.A., Gillis, S., Taylor, C.R. and Rea, T.H. (1984). *In situ* identification of cells in human leprosy granulomas with monoclonal antibodies to interleukin-2 and its receptor. *J. Immunol.*, **132,** 3085–90
35. Rea, T.H., Shen, J-Y. and Modlin, R.L. (1986). Epidermal keratinocyte Ia expression, Langerhans cell hyperplasia and lymphocytic infiltration in skin lesions of leprosy. *Clin. Exp. Immunol.*, **65,** 253–9
36. Wright, D.M., Hirst, R.A. and Waters, M.F.R. (1975). Neural autoantibodies in leprosy. *Lepr. Rev.*, **46,** 157–69
37. Ridley, D.S. (1969). Reactions in leprosy. *Lepr. Rev.*, **40,** 77–81
38. Bjune, G. (1983). Reactions in leprosy. *Lepr. Rev.*, Special Issue 61S-67S
39. Nielson, R., Mshana, R.N., Negesse, Y., Menigistu, G. and Kana, B. (1986). Immunochemical studies of leprous neuritis. *Lepr. Rev.*, **57,** Suppl. 2, 177–87
40. Haregewoin, A., Godal, T., Mustafa, A.S., Belehu, A. and Yemaneberhan, T. (1983). T-cell conditioned media reverse T-cell unresponsiveness in lepromatous leprosy. *Nature (London)*, **303,** 342–4
41. Convit, J., Aranzazu, N., Ulrich, M., Zuñiga, M., Aragon, M.E., Alvarado, J. and Reyes, O. (1983). Investigations related to the development of a leprosy vaccine. *Int. J. Lepr.*, **51,** 531–9
42. Laal, S., Buthani, L.K. and Nath, I. (1985). Natural emergence of antigen-reactive T cells in lepromatous leprosy patients during erythema nodosum leprosum. *Infect. Immun.*, **50,** 887–92
43. Convit, J., Ulrich, M., Aranzazu, N., Castellanos, P.L., Pinardi, M.E. and Reyes, O. (1986). The development of a vaccination model using two microorganisms and its application in leprosy and leishmaniasis. *Lepr. Rev.*, **57,** Suppl. 2, 263–73
44. Convit, J., Avila, J.L., Goihman, M. and Pinardi, M.E. (1972). A test for the

determination of competency in clearing bacilli in leprosy patients. *Bull. WHO*, **46,** 821–6

45. Convit, J., Pinardi, M. E., Rodriguez-Ochoa, G., Ulrich, M., Avila, J. L. and Goihman, M. (1974). Elimination of *Mycobacterium leprae* subsequent to local *in vivo* activation of macrophages in lepromatous leprosy by other mycobacteria. *Clin. Exp. Immunol.*, **17,** 261–5
46. Gross, A., Weiss, E., Tapia, F. J., Aranzazu, N., Gallinotto, M. E. and Convit, J. (1988). Leukocyte subsets in the granulomatous response produced after inoculation with *M. leprae*–BCG in lepromatous patients. *Am. J. Trop. Med. Hyg.*, **38,** 608–12
47. Longley, B. J., Haregewoin, A., de Beaumont, W., Smith, K. A. and Godal, T. (1986). Lepromin stimulates interleukin-2 production and interleukin-2 receptor expression *in situ* in lepromatous leprosy patients. *Lepr. Rev.*, **57,** Suppl. 2, 189–98

3

TUBERCULOSIS OF THE SKIN: CLINICAL ASPECTS

M. HARAHAP

Tuberculosis of the skin is caused by *Mycobacterium tuberculosis* of the human, bovine and, very rarely, the avian type[1]. In man, *M. tuberculosis* and *M. bovis* caused identical skin manifestations. The skin changes elicited by *M. tuberculosis/bovis* infection are polymorphous, depending upon the interplay of host immunity and bacterial virulence.

DEFINITION AND CLASSIFICATION

Tuberculosis of the skin can be divided into the two broad categories of exogenous and endogenous infections[2].

Exogenous infections, arising from direct inoculation with *M. tuberculosis* through a break in the skin, take one of two forms, depending on the immunological status of the individual. If an individual has no previous exposure to mycobacteria, an ulcer appears at the site of entry and is accompanied by lymphadenopathy. Spontaneous resolution of the ulcer within a few weeks is to be expected although disseminated tuberculosis may ensue. The combination of primary cutaneous focus and regional lymphadenopathy forms a primary cutaneous complex or primary inoculation tuberculosis; this type is analogous to the Ghon complex in the lung.

Direct inoculation of tubercle bacilli into the skin of an individual, who is relatively immune to tuberculosis because of previous exposure, causes lesions with an entirely different clinical expression. This exogenous direct inoculation results in tuberculosis verrucosa cutis and lupus vulgaris.

Endogenous infections, which arise from infections elsewhere in the body are: scrofuloderma, produced by contiguous extension from underlying organs; lupus vulgaris, produced by way of the lymphatics or by haematogenous dissemination as in miliary tuberculosis of the skin.

The spread of *M. tuberculosis* from an endogenous source may occur through autoinoculation of mucous membranes and adjoining skin around a bodily orifice, as viable organisms are either expectorated or passed. This condition will lead to tuberculosis cutis orificialis.

A distinction must also be made between a true tuberculous infection of the skin and tuberculids. Tuberculids represent an allergic reaction to haematogenous dissemination of antigen from an internal focus reaching highly immune skin. Mycobacteria cannot be found in tuberculids. Occasional demonstrations of bacilli in tuberculids and positive results from these lesions are attributable to favourable timing in obtaining the tested material and do not contradict the allergic genesis of tuberculids[3]. Histologically most tuberculids exhibit tuberculoid features. A clinical focus of tuberculosis is often present. Tuberculostatics have been found beneficial in tuberculids. However, the tendency to classify a lesion as a tuberculid because of an impressive response to antituberculosis treatment can be misleading, since some tuberculids tend to undergo spontaneous resolution within a relatively short period and, in fact, some cases do not respond to antituberculosis treatment.

In general, the diagnosis of tuberculids rests on:

(1) Lesions which are clinically typical of one of the validated types of tuberculid,

(2) The tuberculid exhibits tuberculoid structure histologically,

(3) A positive tuberculin test,

(4) Previous and concomitant tuberculous focus elsewhere.

A recent clinically relevant classification of tuberculosis of the skin is shown in Table 3.1.

TABLE 3.1 Classification of tuberculosis of the skin

Type	*Mode of infection*	*Tuberculin sensitivity*	*M. tuberculosis in lesions*	*State of immunity*	*Histological caseation*
True tuberculosis of the skin					
Primary inoculation tuberculosis	exogenous inoculation through skin	negative, converting to positive	present	variable, but usually good	considerable
Tuberculosis verrucosa cutis	exogenous inoculation through skin	positive	present	good	moderate
Lupus vulgaris	contiguous extension from nodes, lymphatics; exogenous inoculation; haematogenous	positive	present (with difficulty)	good	variable
Scrofuloderma	contiguous extension underlying infected nodes	positive	present	variable	considerable
Tuberculosis orificialis	autoinoculation of mucous membrane or skin at orifice	positive (negative in advanced stage)	present	poor	considerable
Miliary tuberculosis of the skin	haematogenous	often negative	present	poor	considerable
Tuberculids					
Papulonecrotic tuberculid	haematogenous	positive	absent	good	considerable
Lichen scrofulosorum	haematogenous	positive	absent	good	absent
Erythema induratum	haematogenous	positive	rarely present	good	considerable

EPIDEMIOLOGY

The prevalence of tuberculosis is declining the world over, because of affluence, advanced public health measures, and effective anti-tuberculosis drugs. The incidence of tuberculosis in the USA and Western Europe will continue to decline, although a number of problems lie concealed. Firstly, in areas with large numbers of immigrants from developing countries, tuberculosis will continue to be a problem. Secondly, the changing pattern of tuberculosis shows that there are problem groups in the indigenous population: middle-aged and elderly men, immunocompromised patients, drug addicts, diabetics and patients with AIDS[4]. Thirdly, in some areas tuberculosis has become so uncommon that it may be overlooked[5].

Tuberculosis of the skin is now very rare in the West, but it is still prevalent in some parts of Eastern Europe[6].

Asian immigrants in the USA and Western Europe may exhibit both common and unusual manifestations of cutaneous tuberculosis which may easily be overlooked through lack of familiarity[7].

The incidence of cutaneous tuberculosis versus the total number of outpatients was 0.19% in Korea[8] and 0.065% in Singapore[9]. This disease has recently decreased in both countries as the prevalence of pulmonary tuberculosis has fallen.

Although it has been claimed that cutaneous tuberculosis is rare in the tropics, reports from India suggest that it may not be so uncommon[10]. In other countries in the tropics it is still seen from time to time. The predominant forms of cutaneous tuberculosis in the tropics are scrofuloderma, tuberculosis verrucosa cutis and lupus vulgaris[8–12].

TUBERCULIN TEST

Skin tests are done with Old Tuberculin (OT), which is a filtrate of *M. tuberculosis* culture broth, or with Purified Protein Derivative (PPD), a protein precipitate obtained from filtrates of heat-sterilized cultures of tubercle bacilli. Old Tuberculin (OT) has been replaced by Purified Protein Derivative (PPD). Preparations are standardized in terms of biological reactivity as tuberculin units (TU). Although multiple puncture methods (Heaf test) are often used for testing children, the Mantoux method, which uses 5 TU of PPD is the best way to identify tuberculous infection.

The tuberculin test is performed in the volar surface of the forearm with a 1 ml tuberculin syringe. The initial test dose most commonly used is 5 TU in 0.1 ml. Higher doses are injected when test with a lower dose was negative. Only 1 TU is given to individuals suspected of extreme hypersensitivity.

The test is interpreted by measuring the diameter of induration as detected by gentle palpation 48–72 h after injection. An induration of

10 mm or greater is a positive reaction indicating individuals who have been infected with tuberculosis, but does not distinguish between the presence of active disease and past infection, nor does it denote immunity to tuberculosis. This distinction must be made on clinical and laboratory findings. The chief value of the test lies in exclusion. If negative, it can be fairly concluded that the patient does not have active tuberculosis, with the exceptions noted below.

Both false-positive and false-negative tuberculin reactions occur. False-positive reactions may result from infections with non-tuberculous mycobacteria, which may cause a lower grade tuberculin sensitization that usually produces reactions smaller than 10 mm. False-negative reactions occur in patients with malnutrition; during the course of certain current infections, especially measles and influenza; late in the course of pregnancy; miliary tuberculosis, sarcoidosis, Hodgkin's disease or in persons receiving corticosteroids or immunosuppressive drugs.

Individuals immunized with attenuated tubercle bacilli (BCG) will become tuberculin-positive. However, the dermal reaction to PPD is usually not as large as that which follows natural infection, usually does not persist as long, and varies from strain to strain of vaccine.

IMMUNIZATION WITH BCG (BACILLE CALMETTE GUÉRIN)

BCG (Bacille Calmette Guérin) is an attenuated strain of *M. bovis* developed by Calmette and Guérin which has been given to hundreds of millions of persons as a vaccine against tuberculosis. Artificial infection with the organism stimulates the immunological response as occurring with natural tuberculous infection. Thus, BCG vaccination affords 30–80% protection against the development of tuberculosis in susceptible and appropriate populations. No protection is provided for persons who are already infected. BCG vaccination does not prevent an infection with tubercle bacilli from actually taking place but its effect is rather to prevent the bacilli from multiplying at such a rate that they result in disease. It should therefore be most effective in persons who are infected with virulent tubercle bacilli soon after getting vaccinated.

The reported effectiveness of BCG vaccination has been clearly demonstrated in several controlled studies, but appears to vary in different communities. The protective efficacy of BCG vaccination in different countries of the world has varied from about 60–80% in the UK[13,14] to 0% in the Southern USA and South India[15]. Unsatisfactory results from BCG vaccination have been reported most often from communities where non-tuberculous mycobacteria are common. These non-tuberculous infections convey some protection against tuberculosis: BCG vaccination to these already partly immune subjects blunts the effect of BCG. Other factors that may be responsible for the low efficacy include variations in the potency of different strains of the organisms and differing conditions and methods of administration of the vaccine, and poor nutritional status and unfavourable genetic factors in the vaccinated persons.

Even in those studies where no protection is observed, the disseminated forms of tuberculosis which have such high mortalities among children were virtually eliminated. Mass BCG vaccination in developing countries must be given before infection has taken place, preferably at birth or in infancy. In communities where this BCG campaign has been efficiently implemented, the mortality and morbidity from tuberculosis in childhood have fallen greatly.

In countries where the prevalence of tuberculosis is low, BCG vaccination is indicated for:

(1) Certain high-risk groups, such as medical students, doctors, nurses, laboratory workers and other hospital workers;

(2) Contacts, e.g. babies of infected mothers, etc.;

(3) Travellers to high prevalence areas.

In developed countries subjects for BCG are first tuberculin tested using the Mantoux test or the Heaf-multiple puncture technique. However, in developing countries, where the prevalence of tuberculosis is not low, BCG has been given indiscriminately without previous tuberculin tests, and WHO advocates this direct and universal vaccination because preliminary tuberculin tests would considerably reduce the numbers of people returning for BCG.

DERMATOLOGICAL COMPLICATIONS OF BCG VACCINATION

The clinical course of a normal BCG vaccination is a papule, becoming an indurated nodule in 12 weeks. A small ulcer may occur at the site of injection, and then slowly heals, leaving a scar.

Conversion usually takes place in 3–12 weeks after vaccination. If a subject has previously been infected but with a negative tuberculin test, BCG vaccination may provoke an accelerated reaction. The regional lymph nodes may enlarge but usually heal without breaking down.

Large ulcers or abscesses are seen when BCG is injected too deeply. Lymphadenitis may occur, particularly in infants and in the younger age groups.

Adverse reactions to BCG are very rare in comparison to the great number of vaccinations carried out.

Non-specific complications include keloid formation, which occurs preferentially on the upper outer arm, urticaria and erythema multiforme. Unusual reactions have included generalized haemorrhagic rashes or maculopapular eruptions.

Specific complications arising from BCG vaccination comprise tuberculous processes caused by the BCG organism. Lupus vulgaris, scrofuloderma, tuberculids, tuberculosis verrucosa cutis and generalized adenitis may occur[16]. In immunodeficient patients, especially children, and in immunodepressed patients, disseminated BCG infections may occur.

Systemic reaction, such as anaphylaxis, and a syndrome resembling tuberculin shock may be fatal.

DIAGNOSIS

Primary inoculation tuberculosis

This is a primary infection in an individual previously free of tuberculosis in any form. The disease usually occurs in infants and children, although occasionally in adults with a prior negative tuberculin test.

An ulcer occurs at the inoculation site and the regional lymph nodes become painful, tender and enlarged. Bacilli are numerous in both the ulcer and its satellite lymph nodes. It is usually found on the face or extremities. Systemic symptoms are minimal or absent. The primary tuberculous lesion usually heals after a few months but the enlarged glands may persist and break down.

A case of primary cutaneous inoculation tuberculosis has been reported secondary to 'Jail tattooing'[17] and in another case this type of cutaneous tuberculosis appeared on the vaginal mucosa, probably due to inoculation during sexual contact[18].

The demonstration of *M. tuberculosis* in suspected lesions with Ziehl–Neelsen stain, its successful culture, and proof of its virulence in guinea pigs confirm the diagnosis.

Histologically, in the early stages there is non-specific inflammation with necrosis and ulceration. After 4 weeks the infiltrate changes to a more distinct tuberculoid appearance with lymphocytes, epithelioid cells and Langhans giant cells. Typical caseation necrosis becomes evident. Acid-fast bacilli may be demonstrable[19,20].

Coccidioidomycosis, blastomycosis, syphilis, leishmaniasis, yaws, tularemia and atypical mycobacterial disease may resemble primary inoculation tuberculosis. These conditions can be readily excluded by skin biopsies, cultures, tissue smears, serological studies and historical and physical findings.

Tuberculosis verrucosa cutis

Most cases are due to an exogenous reinfection in individuals with marked cutaneous hypersensitivity and good immunity. The lesions start usually as indurated, circumscribed red-brown warty plaques. They may be single or multiple, gradually increase in number and coalesce to form verrucous plaques of coin or palm size, or even much larger (Figures 3.1–3.3). The most frequent sites are the dorsal surfaces of the feet, hands, knees and buttocks[21].

A 33-year-old lesion of tuberculosis verrucosa cutis with liver involvement has been observed in a male peasant. The association of tuberculosis verrucosa cutis with visceral involvement has often been reported, the visceral lesions usually being the origin of the cutaneous lesion. It may happen, as in this case, that the visceral lesions originate from the cutaneous ones since we are dealing with bacilliferous lesions[22].

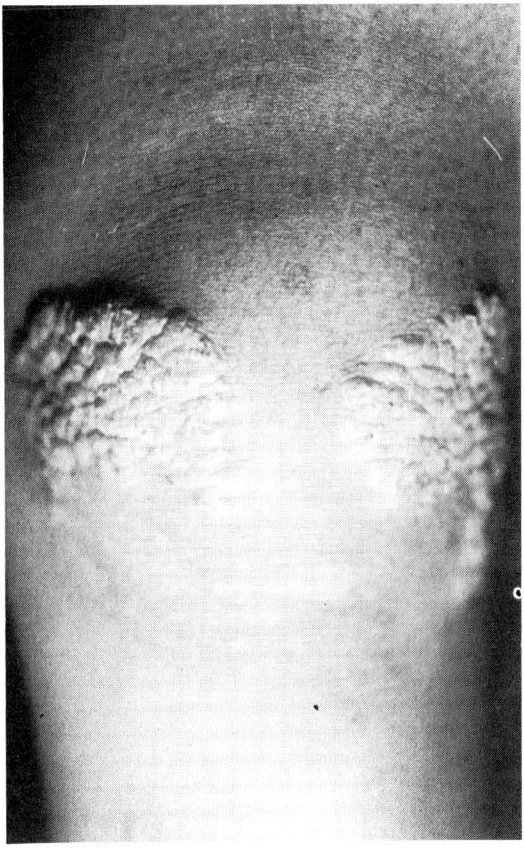

FIGURE 3.1 Tuberculosis verrucosa cutis on the knee. Circumscribed red-brown warty plaques

The histological picture shows hyperkeratosis, papillomatosis and acanthosis. Tuberculoid structures with a moderate amount of necrosis are seen. There may be caseation necrosis. Tubercle bacilli are present[23].

This type of skin tuberculosis must be differentiated from cases of atypical mycobacterial granuloma, sporotrichosis, chromomycosis, tinea profunda (Majocchi's granuloma), verrucous epidermal nevus and even verruca vulgaris.

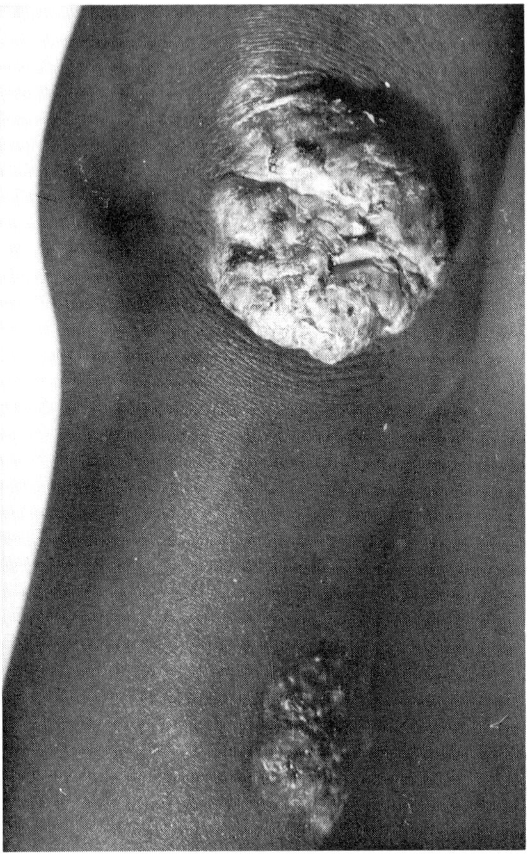

FIGURE 3.2 Tuberculosis verrucosa cutis on the knee

Lupus vulgaris

Lupus vulgaris occurs in individuals with immunity induced by previous tuberculous infection.

It is most prevalent on exposed parts, especially the face. It can be located on the extremities, and involvement of the trunk is rare. The bacilli come to the skin from the nose or from other active foci of tuberculosis through haematogenous routes or by contiguity.

The individual lesion is a small nodule, characterized by a reddish brown colour, which, when pressed against a thin piece of glass slide,

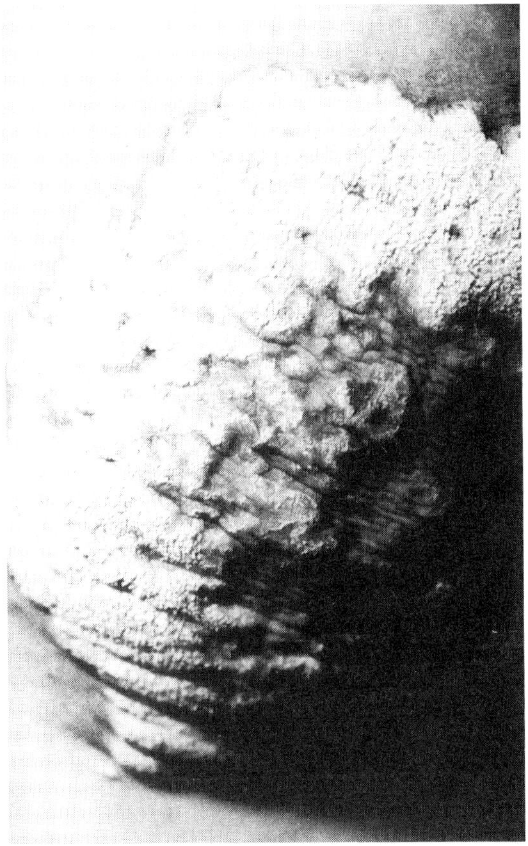

FIGURE 3.3 Tuberculosis verrucosa cutis. Hyperkeratotic plaque

has a pale brownish-yellow or 'apple-jelly' colour. The disease causes ulceration, and on involution leaves deforming scars. Typical apple-jelly nodules with scarring are distinctive[21] (Figures 3.4–3.8).

The oral cavity is an unusual site of lupus vulgaris. Four cases have been reported in patients with asymptomatic pulmonary tuberculosis[24].

Histologically, tubercles or tuberculoid structures composed of epithelioid cells and giant cells are present. Acid-fast bacilli are almost never found in microscopic sections. Caseation necrosis within the tubercles is only slight or may be absent. Secondary changes in the

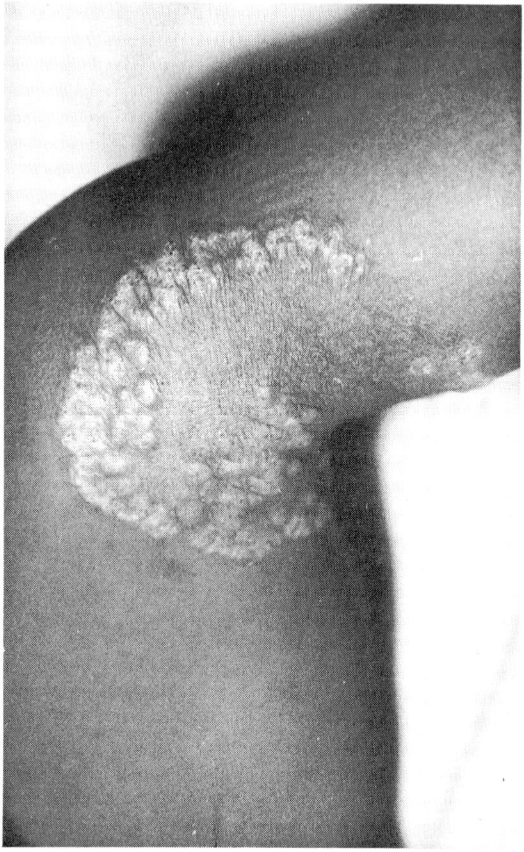

FIGURE 3.4 Lupus vulgaris with typical apple-jelly nodules

epidermis are common, sometimes flattened and other times hypertrophic[19].

The differential diagnosis includes acne vulgaris and rosacea. Papular syphilids are monomorphic and bilateral, and spirochaetes may be demonstrated in the serum from the lesion. Lupus erythematosus may simulate lupus vulgaris, but the presence of apple-jelly nodules and skin biopsy eliminates lupus erythematosus.

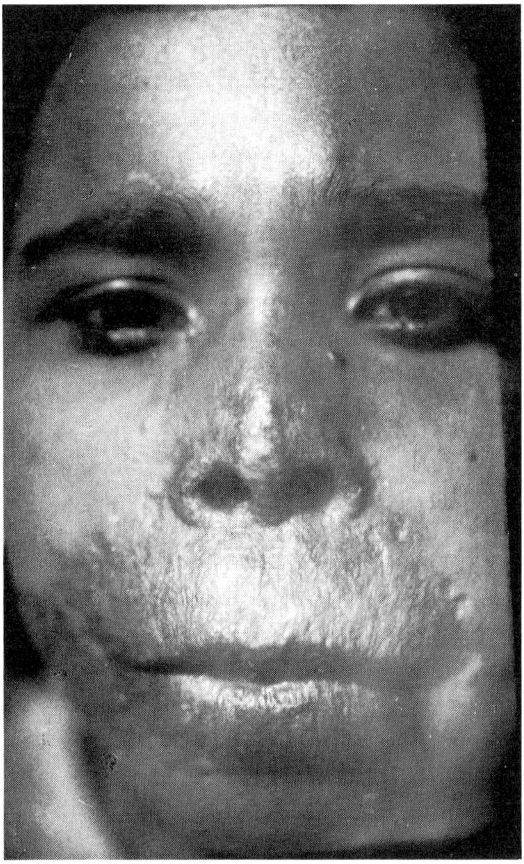

FIGURE 3.5 Lupus vulgaris around the mouth. On involution leaves scar

Scrofuloderma

Scrofuloderma involves the skin by direct extension, usually secondary to underlying tuberculous lymph nodes, bones or joints. The nodules and gummata appear over the lymph nodes of the neck, sternal region, knees or ankles. The process usually begins with a deep, purplish induration of the skin overlying tuberculous lymphatic glands, but caseation soon makes them fluctuant. The glands tend to break down and form ulcers that serve as draining sinuses, which discharge purulent and caseous exudate. Chronic discharging sinuses and ulcerations

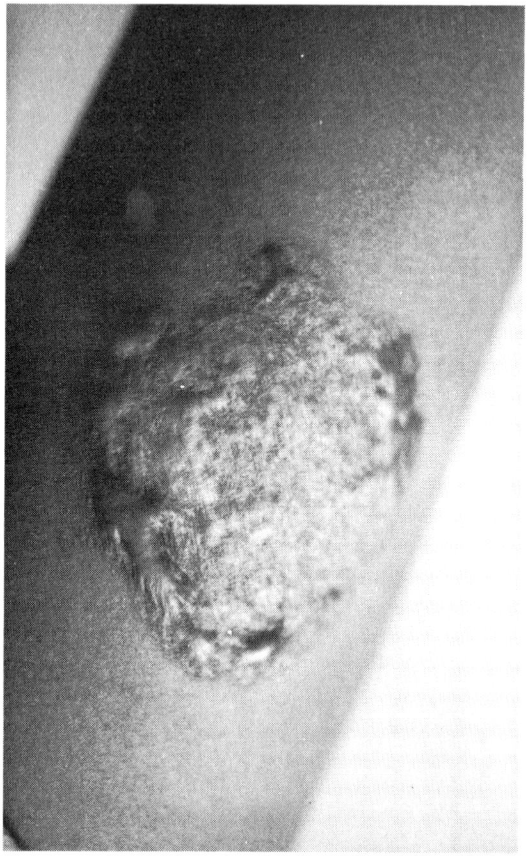

FIGURE 3.6 Lupus vulgaris on the arm

are sometimes confluent and healing is by hypertrophic or cord-like cicatrices[21] (Figure 3.9).

The histological picture shows non-specific changes, such as abscess formation or ulceration. In the deep cutis one usually sees caseation necrosis and formation of cavity filled with liquefied debris, the walls of the cavity being formed by tuberculous granulation tissue. Usually the tubercle bacilli can be detected in histological sections[19,20].

Lesions of syphilitic gumma, sporotrichosis, blastomycosis, actinomycosis, pyogenic lymphadenitis and lymphogranuloma venereum may be similar clinically. These conditions can be excluded by sero-

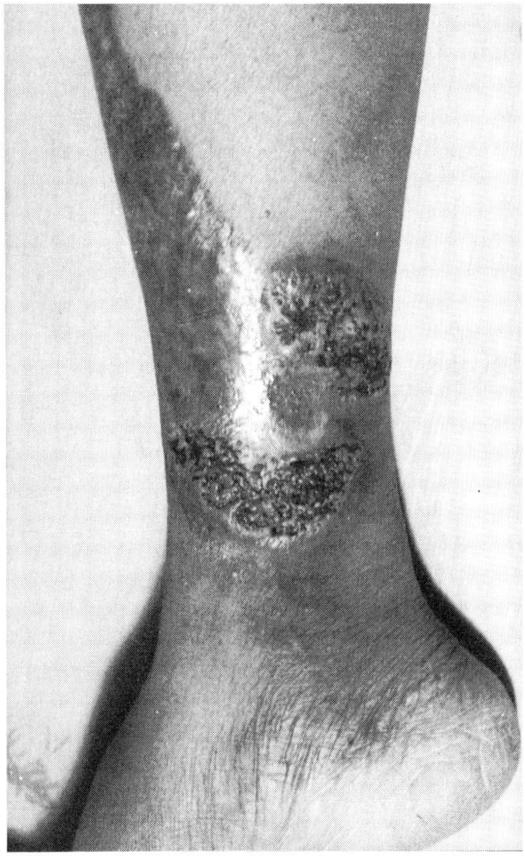

FIGURE 3.7 Ulcerative lupus vulgaris on the leg

logical studies, cultures, skin biopsies, tissue smears and historical and physical findings.

Tuberculosis orificialis

This form of localized tuberculosis occurs at the mucocutaneous borders of the nose, mouth, anus, urinary meatus and vagina, due to autoinoculation of mycobacteria from severe visceral tuberculosis, and with failing resistance to the disease.

Erythema induratum

Erythema induratum usually occurs in young women who have glandular tuberculosis and acrocyanosis. Tuberculin sensitivity is marked. The lower calf is the preferred site and lesions rarely occur on the front of the leg. The lesions are soft recurrent nodules, usually symmetrical and indolent. The nodules usually persist for 3 or 4 months and eventually ulcerate. The ulcers have irregular shapes and are deeply excavated with undermined edges.

Histologically, there are vascular changes characterized by general thickening of the veins and arteries, endothelial proliferation of the intima with obliteration, thrombus formation and necrosis. The presence of epithelioid cell tubercles and caseation necrosis favours the diagnosis of erythema induratum[19,23].

Erythema induratum should be differentiated from erythema nodosum, nodular allergic vasculitis, gummatous syphilis and the nodose lesions due to iodides and bromides. Erythema nodosum affects chiefly the shins and produces tender red nodules that do not ulcerate. Syphilitic gummata tend to be more chronic and occur asymmetrically in older people with positive serological tests. Nodular allergic vasculitis, iododerma and bromoderma can be excluded by skin biopsy findings, a history of halide ingestion and the presence of elevated serum bromide.

It is believed that erythema induratum responds better to corticosteroids than to antituberculosis drugs.

THE SPECTRUM OF IMMUNE RESPONSES OF CUTANEOUS TUBERCULOSIS

Differences in cell-mediated immunity and a spectrum of immune responses have been demonstrated in many diseases such as leprosy, leishmaniasis and syphilis[27]. Clinical, morphological and immunological studies enabled the spectrum of human tuberculosis to be determined.

Lenzini *et al.*[28] demonstrated that tuberculosis can be classified into two polar groups: the first group showing good cell-mediated immunity and little or no antibody formation and the second group poor cellular responses and excessive antibody production.

Different types of cutaneous tuberculosis seemed to form a continuous spectrum of immune responses; at one end by scrofuloderma and at another by lupus vulgaris. Tuberculosis verrucosa cutis probably occupies a position in between[10].

MYCOBACTERIAL SKIN INFECTION IN PATIENTS WITH ACQUIRED IMMUNODEFICIENCY SYNDROME

Mycobacterial disease is common among patients with AIDS[29–31]. The most frequently isolated cause is *Mycobacterium avium* complex, but in some groups in which tuberculous infection is highly prevalent, *M. tuberculosis* is more common[32,33].

Disseminated tuberculosis has been frequently reported in patients with AIDS, especially in some groups, such as Haitians and intravenous drug users[34,35]. Scrofuloderma has been reported in a patient with AIDS[36,37]. Ill-defined macular, discoloured lesions on the forearms caused by *Mycobacterium avium-intracellulare* have been reported in patients with acquired immunodeficiency syndrome[38].

Mycobacterium marinum has been isolated from ecthymatous lesions of another patient[39].

Available data indicate that extrapulmonary forms of tuberculosis, particularly lymphatic and disseminated (miliary), are seen much more frequently among patients with human immunodeficiency virus (HIV) infection than among patients without such infection. It is recommended that initial treatment of tuberculosis in these cases include at least three standard antituberculosis drugs for a minimum of 9 months[40].

TREATMENT

The modern treatment of tuberculosis is based on the administration of effective chemotherapy. The aims of therapy are not only to cure patients, but also to avoid relapse, and to prevent the emergence of drug-resistant mutants. Treatment regimens do not differ for pulmonary and extrapulmonary tuberculosis[41].

The antituberculosis drugs

The first-line drugs used for previously untreated disease are isoniazid, rifampin, streptomycin, pyrazinamide, ethambutol, thioacetazone and p-amino salicylic acid (PAS). They represent the first choice because of their effectiveness, relatively low toxicity, and relatively low cost. The second-line drugs, which may be used in treating patients whose first-line treatment has failed, are ethionamide or prothionamide, cycloserine, kanamycin, capreomycin and viomycin. In general, the second-line drugs are less effective, more toxic and more expensive than the first-line drugs. Chemotherapeutic regimens for the treatment of tuberculosis[42] are as follows.

Daily long-term regimens

An *initial phase* using at least three drugs: isoniazid (adults up to 300 mg daily; children 6 mg/kg daily), is given with a companion drug, which may be ethambutol (adults 15 mg/kg daily; children 25 mg/kg daily), rifampin (adults 450–600 mg daily; children 20 mg/kg daily), PAS (adults 10–15 g daily; children 300 mg/kg daily) or thioacetazone (adults 150 mg daily; children 4 mg/kg daily) and a third drug: streptomycin (adults 0.75–1 g daily; children 20 mg/kg daily). This initial phase of three-drug chemotherapy is given for 1–3 months. The *continuation phase* consists usually of two drugs: isoniazid and a companion drug, which may be ethambutol or rifampin (in developed countries) and is continued for 12–18 months. In developing countries PAS or thioacetazone is generally administered as a companion drug because both are cheap.

Intermittent supervised chemotherapy

The intermittent regimens can far more easily be administered under direct supervision on an outpatient basis than daily regimens. Streptomycin (1 g daily) is injected twice weekly with orally high dosage (15 mg/kg) isoniazid. Treatment should continue for at least 18 months.

Short-course chemotherapy

In developed countries, a daily regimen is currently recommended of isoniazid (5–10 mg/kg daily up to 300 mg/day p.o.) and rifampin (10–20 mg/kg daily up to 600 mg/day p.o.) for 9 months, usually supplemented with ethambutol (15–25 mg/kg daily p.o.), streptomycin (15–20 mg/kg daily up to 1 g/day i.m.) or pyrazinamide (15–30 mg/kg daily p.o.) for a 2–3-months initial phase.

This regimen containing all three of the drugs, isoniazid, rifampin, and pyrazinamide, is highly effective for patients with initially resistant infection.

A 6-month regimen of chemotherapy is acceptable if four drugs (isoniazid, rifampin, pyrazinamide, and streptomycin or ethambutol) are administered for 2 months and are followed by an additional 4 months of isoniazid and rifampin, with all drugs given under close supervision[41]. The administration of pyridoxine (50 mg/day p.o.) prevents complications of peripheral neuritis and nervous system disorders.

Developing countries

In developing countries the choice of regimen is often determined primarily by the cost. Several possible schedules are listed below:

(1) A direct supervised regimen based on a 3-month initial daily phase followed by a twice-weekly isoniazid (300 mg) and streptomycin (0.75–1 g).

(2) An 8-month regimen of daily streptomycin (0.75–1 g), isoniazid (300 mg), rifampin (600 mg) and pyrazinamide (1.5–2 g) for 1 month followed by twice-weekly streptomycin, isoniazid and pyrazinamide is also not costly.

(3) A complete oral regimen of ethambutol (15 mg/kg), isoniazid (300 mg), rifampin (600 mg), and pyrazinamide (1.5–2 g), three times a week for 6 months is also effective, but costs more.

(4) An 8-month regimen of streptomycin, isoniazid, rifampin and

pyrazinamide for 2 months followed by isoniazid and thioacetazone is not expensive. Patients tolerate thioacetazone poorly.

Other treatment

Small lesions of lupus vulgaris or warty tuberculosis may be excised, but chemotherapy should also be given. Plastic surgery may help to repair the disfigurement caused by long-standing lupus vulgaris.

ACKNOWLEDGEMENT

Figures are reproduced with permission of the Department of Dermatology, University of Indonesia Medical School, Jakarta, Indonesia.

REFERENCES

1. Christiansen, J. V. (1968). Lupus vulgaris gigantea caused by *Mycobacterium avium*. In Jadassohn, W. and Schirren, C. G. (eds.) *Proceedings of the 13th International Congress of Dermatology*. Vol. II, pp. 1319–20. (Berlin: Springer Verlag)
2. Beyt, B. E., Orthbals, D. W., Cruz, D. J. S., Kobayashi, G., Eisen, A. Z. and Medoff, G. (1981). Cutaneous Mycobacteriosis: analysis of 34 cases with a new classification of the disease. *Medicine*, **60**, 95–109
3. Wise, F. and Satenstein, D. L. (1921). Clinical and histologic features of certain types of cutaneous tuberculosis. *Arch. Derm. Syph.*, **4**, 586–608
4. James, D. G. and Mishra, B. B. (1984). The changing pattern of tuberculosis. *Postgrad. Med. J.*, **60**, 92–7
5. McNicol, M. (1983). Trends in the epidemiology of tuberculosis – a physician's view. *J. Clin. Pathol.*, **36**, 1087–90
6. Dinning, W. J. and Marston, S. (1985). Cutaneous and ocular tuberculosis: a review. *J. R. Soc. Med.*, **78**, 576–81
7. Hetzel, M. R. and Williams, I. P. (1979). Cutaneous tuberculosis in an Asian. *Pract. Med.*, **223**, 563–4
8. Kim, Y. P. and Sohn, H. S. (1978). Cutaneous tuberculosis in Korea. *Proceedings of the Third Regional Conference of Dermatology*. Den Pasar Bali, Indonesia, November, pp. 499–513 (Indonesian Society of Dermatology and Venereology)
9. Goh, Y. S., Ong, B. H. and Rajan, V. S. (1974). Tuberculosis cutis in Singapore: a two year experience. *Singapore Med. J.*, **15**, 223–6
10. Sehgal, V. N., Srivastava, G., Khurana, V. K., Sharma, V. K., Bhalla, P. and

Beohar, P. C. (1987). An appraisal of epidemiologic, clinical, bacteriologic, histopathologic, and immunologic parameters in cutaneous tuberculosis. *Int. J. Dermatol.*, **26,** 521–6

11. Wirjohatmodjo, N. T., Djuanda, A., Wiryadi, B. E. and Wirawan, R. (1978). Multiple tuberculosis cutis (lupus vulgaris or tuberculosis verrucosa cutis). *Proceedings of the Third Regional Conference of Dermatology*, Den Pasar Bali, Indonesia, November, pp. 518–22 (Indonesian Society of Dermatology and Venereology)
12. Wong, K. O., Lee, K. P. and Chin, S. F. (1968). Tuberculosis of the skin in Hong Kong (a review of 160 cases). *Br. J. Dermatol.*, **80,** 287–92
13. Great Britain Medical Research Council (1972). BCG and vole bacillus vaccines in the prevention of tuberculosis in adolescence and early adult life. *Bull. WHO*, **46,** 371
14. Capewell, S., France, A., Uzel, N. and Leitch, A. G. (1986). The current value of tuberculin testing and BCG vaccination in school children. *Br. J. Dis. Chest*, **80,** 254–64
15. Tuberculosis Prevention Trial, Madras (1979). Trial of BCG vaccines in South India for tuberculosis prevention. First report. *Bull. WHO*, **57,** 819
16. Dostrovsky, A. and Sagher, F. (1963). Dermatological complications of BCG vaccination. *Br. J. Dermatol.*, **75,** 181–92
17. Horney, D. A., Gaither, J. M., Lauer, R., Norins, A. L. and Mathur, P. N. (1985). Cutaneous inoculation tuberculosis secondary to 'Jailhouse tattooing'. *Arch. Dermatol.*, **121,** 648–50
18. Blondeel, A., Masson, Th. and Wilkin, P. (1982). Chancre tuberculeux d'inoculation a transmission sexuelle. *Dermatologica*, **165,** 398–400
19. Lever, W. F. and Schaumburg-Lever, G. (1983). *Histopathology of the Skin*. pp. 297–303. (Philadelphia: Lippincott)
20. Montgomery, H. (1937). Histopathology of various types of cutaneous tuberculosis. *Arch. Dermatol. Syph.*, **35,** 698–715
21. Harahap, M. (1983). Tuberculosis of the skin. *Int. J. Dermatol.*, **22,** 542–5
22. Bordalo, O. and Silva, G. E. (1987). Tuberculosis verrucosa cutis with liver involvement. *Clin. Exp. Dermatol.*, **12,** 283–5
23. Hirsh, B. C. and Johnson, W. C. (1984). Pathology of granulomatous diseases. Epithelioid granulomas. Part 1. *Int. J. Dermatol.*, **23,** 237–46
24. Laskaris, G. C. and Nicolis, G. D. (1981). Lupus vulgaris of the oral mucosa. *Dermatologica*, **162,** 183–90
25. Frix, C. D. and Bronson, D. M. (1986). Acute miliary tuberculosis in a child with anhidrotic ectodermal dysplasia. *Pediatr. Dermatol.*, **3,** 464–7
26. Wilson-Jones, E. and Winkelmann, R. K. (1986). Papulonecrotic tuberculid: a neglected disease in Western countries. *J. Am. Acad. Dermatol.*, **14,** 815–26
27. WHO Scientific Group Report (1973). Cell-mediated immunity and resistance to infection. *WHO Tech. Rep. Ser. Geneva*, 519
28. Lenzini, L., Rottoli, P. and Rottoli, L. (1977). The spectrum of human tuberculosis. *Clin. Exp. Immunol.*, **27,** 230–7
29. Wong, B., Edwards, F. F., Kiehn, T. E. *et al.* (1985). Continuous high-grade *Mycobacterium avium intracellulare* bacteremia in patients with the acquired immunodeficiency syndrome. *Am. J. Med.*, **78,** 35–40
30. Macher, A. M., Kovacs, J. A., Gill, V. *et al.* (1983). Bacteremia due to *Mycobacterium avium intracellulare* in the acquired immunodeficiency syndrome. *Ann. Intern. Med.*, **99,** 782–5

31. Eng, R. H., Forrester, C., Smith, S. M. and Sobel, H. (1984). *Mycobacterium xenopi* infection in a patient with immunodeficiency syndrome. *Chest*, **86,** 145–7
32. Pape, J. W., Liautaud, B., Thomas, F. *et al.* (1983). Characteristics of the acquired immunodeficiency syndrome (AIDS) in Haiti. *N. Engl. J. Med.*, **309,** 945–50
33. Maayan, S., Wormser, G. P., Hewlett, D. *et al.* (1985). Acquired immunodeficiency syndrome (AIDS) in an economically disadvantaged population. *Arch. Intern. Med.*, **145,** 1607–12
34. Zakowski, P., Fligiel, S., Berlin, O. G. W. *et al.* (1982). Disseminated *Mycobacterium avium* in homosexual men dying of acquired immunodeficiency. *J. Am. Med. Assoc.*, **248,** 2980–2
35. de la Loma, A., Manrique, A., Rubrio, R. *et al.* (1985). Generalized tuberculosis in a patient with acquired immunodeficiency syndrome. *J. Infect.*, **10,** 57–9
36. Marchiando, A. (1984). Scrofula followed by AIDS (letter). *Ear Nose Throat J.*, **63,** 197–8
37. Penneys, N. S. and Hicks, B. (1985). Unusual cutaneous lesions associated with acquired immunodeficiency syndrome. *J. Am. Acad. Dermatol.*, **13,** 845–52
38. Pitchenik, A. E., Cole, C., Russell, B. W. *et al.* (1984). Tuberculosis, atypical mycobacteriosis, and the acquired immunodeficiency syndrome among Haitian and non-Haitian patients in South Florida. *Ann. Intern. Med.*, **101,** 641–5
39. Kaplan, M. H., Sadick, N., McNutt, N. S. *et al.* (1987). Dermatologic findings and manifestations of acquired immunodeficiency syndrome (AIDS). *J. Am. Acad. Dermatol.*, **16,** 485–506
40. Centers for Disease Control (1987). Diagnosis and Management of Mycobacterial infection and disease in persons with Human Immunodeficiency Virus infection. *Ann. Intern. Med.*, **106,** 254–6
41. Corsella, B. F. (1987). New approach to treatment of pulmonary and extrapulmonary tuberculosis. Possible ramifications of cutaneous Mycobacterial infections. *Int. J. Dermatol.*, **26,** 185–9
42. Stead, W. W. and Dutt, A. K. (1982). Chemotherapy for tuberculosis today. *Am. Rev. Respir. Dis.*, **125,** 94–101

4

ENVIRONMENTAL (ATYPICAL) MYCOBACTERIA: CLINICAL ASPECTS

K. J. TOMECKI

Few people would dispute the importance of the genus *Mycobacteria* as a source of human disease. Throughout history, the entire genus has produced important disease with significant morbidity and mortality – tuberculosis, leprosy, Buruli ulcers and, most recently, opportunistic and fatal infections in AIDS. Understandably, *Mycobacteria tuberculosis* and *Mycobacteria leprae*, two obligate human pathogens, are probably still the most important representatives of the genus and command most of the attention. Mycobacteria other than *M. tuberculosis* and *M. leprae* often produce human disease. In contrast to the decreasing incidence of tuberculosis, the incidence of disease produced by these non-tuberculous, non-lepromatous mycobacteria continues to rise in the western hemisphere[1]. Still inappropriately called 'anonymous', 'atypical', etc., these environmental mycobacteria – ubiquitous, saprophytic organisms present throughout nature – are more representative of the genus than their more famous cousins. Environmental mycobacteria is a more accurate term for those non-tuberculous, non-lepromatous mycobacteria that exist in nature.

EPIDEMIOLOGY

The environmental mycobacteria contain hundreds of species, most of which are widely distributed in nature. Frequent contact with these organisms is inevitable. Excluding *M. tuberculosis* and *M. leprae*, there are now approximately 50 species of these mycobacteria capable of infecting man and woman. The organisms are sturdy, resilient acid-fast bacilli that are structurally similar to *M. tuberculosis* and *M. bovis* and are biologically different from *M. tuberculosis, M. bovis* and *M. leprae*. Environmental mycobacteria exist throughout the environment, particularly where water meets the soil – lakes, ponds, swamps, rivers, pools, etc.; they have contaminated hospital water supplies[2] and natural water sources[3]. Water is an obvious and important reservoir[4], especially for two species, *M. marinum* and *M. xenopi*.

Humans frequently have contact with these commensal organisms of low virulence. Organisms often contaminate sputum, urine and gastric juices, usually without sequelae or resultant disease, and isolation of one of these organisms does not imply the presence of disease. To establish a link between one of these organisms and disease, the following should occur: regular retrieval of the organism (more than two occasions), preferably from a sterile source; heavy concentration of the recovered organism; documented granulomatous disease consistent with infection and the clinical presentation of the patient.

Unlike tuberculosis, there is no evidence for transmission of disease between humans or between animals and humans. These organisms have no known vector, and, except for *M. smegmatis*, they are not part of normal human flora.

MICROBIOLOGY

The Runyon classification is still a valid and reasonable way to categorize and understand the environmental mycobacteria[5]. Developed in 1959, the classification uses rate of growth and pigment production to separate the environmental mycobacteria into four groups (Table 4.1).

TABLE 4.1 Environmental mycobacteria. Runyon classification

Group	*Name*	*Pigment*	*Growth*
I	photochromogens	yellow	2–3 weeks
II	scotochromogens	yellow/orange	2–3 weeks
III	non-chromogens	none	2–3 weeks
IV	rapid growers	variable	3–5 days

Group I *photochromogens,* slow growing mycobacteria that produce pigment after exposure to light

Group II *scotochromogens,* slow growing mycobacteria that produce pigment in the dark

Group III *non-chromogens,* slow growing mycobacteria that produce no pigment with or without exposure to light

Group IV *rapid growers,* fast growing mycobacteria that usually produce no pigment, but may

Slow growing mycobacteria exhibit growth within 2–3 weeks; rapid growing mycobacteria exhibit growth within 3–5 days. Slight variations in pigment occur occasionally.

Environmental mycobacteria grow well on Löwenstein–Jensen media, a standard growth media for acid-fast bacilii. *M. fortuitum* and *M. chelonae*, two rapid growers, grow quickly on blood agar and chocolate agar[6]; they also grow on Sauton agar, in contrast to slow growing organisms which do not[7]. Most environmental mycobacteria grow very well at 35–37°C except for *M. marinum* and *M. ulcerans* which grow readily at 30–32°C and *M. xenopi* which grows better at 45°C.

Several biochemical tests can help to identify accurately individual environmental mycobacteria. Of the available tests the niacin test and the nitrate reduction test easily separate *M. tuberculosis* from the environmental mycobacteria. These tests are positive for *M. tuberculosis* and uniformly negative for most of the environmental mycobacteria. *In vitro* drug susceptibility testing, important in determining treatment of disease, allows rough placement of an organism into a

Runyon group. *M. tuberculosis* and organisms in Group I are usually sensitive to most antituberculous drugs. *M. marinum* and *M. kansasii*, Group I organisms, are usually sensitive to rifampin, ethambutol, and ethionamide. Organisms in Group IV are invariably resistant to the same drugs. Organisms in Group II and III have variable and unpredicted sensitivity to the same drugs. Infections with *M. avium–intracellulare–scrofulaceum* (*MAIS*), an important pathogen in AIDS, typically show *in vitro* resistance to standard antituberculous drugs.

In contrast to tuberculosis, skin tests with prepared antigens from the environmental mycobacteria are useless in the evaluation of patients infected with one of the environmental mycobacteria.

CLINICAL DISEASE

The primary pathogens of each Runyon group and the organs commonly affected are:

Group I	*M. marinum* (skin); *M. kansasii* (lungs)
Group II	*M. scrofulaceum* (lymph nodes)
Group III	*M. avium–intracellulare,* now termed MAIS (as a complex) with inclusion of *M. scrofulaceum* (lungs)
Group IV	*M. fortuitum* and *M. chelonae* (skin)

Most of the environmental mycobacteria never produce human disease. The most common human pathogens are *M. kansasii, MAIS, M. scrofulaceum, M. ulcerans, M. marinum, M. fortuitum* and *M. chelonae* (Table 4.2). Pulmonary disease in adults accounts for the

TABLE 4.2 Environmental mycobacteria. Common human pathogens

Skin	*M. marinum* *M. fortuitum* *M. chelonae* *M. ulcerans*
Lungs	*MAIS* *M. kansasii*
Lymph nodes	*MAIS* *M. scrofulaceum*

vast majority of infection produced by the environmental mycobacteria[8]. *M. kansasii* and *MAIS* are the major pulmonary pathogens and tend to produce chronic pulmonary disease in patients with predisposing factors such as chronic obstructive pulmonary disease, pre-existing lung disease, healed pulmonary tuberculosis, AIDS, immunosuppression[1,4,9]. *MAIS*, an infrequent pathogen before the advent of AIDS, now commonly invades the lungs and bone marrow of AIDS patients. *M. kansasii* and *MAIS* rarely produce pulmonary disease in children[8], except for *MAIS* in AIDS patients. Cervical adenitis, usually caused by *MAIS*, is the most common presentation of disease in children[8] and tends to occur more commonly in children not vaccinated with BCG[8].

Immunocompromised patients are at the highest risk for infection with the environmental mycobacteria[9], especially disseminated disease with *MAIS* as the predominant pathogen[10]. Treatment for disseminated *MAIS* infection in such patients is difficult and often requires involved therapy with five or more drugs[10]. In contrast, disseminated *MAIS* infection still occurs mainly in children with normal immunity[9]. This presentation will probably change as AIDS continues to affect more people.

When environmental mycobacteria produce skin disease one of two scenarios usually occurs[6]:

(1) Infection of a normal host, usually after trauma or surgery, with subsequent development of cellulitis or an abscess 4–6 weeks after inoculation;

(2) Infection of an immunocompromised host with subsequent development of several subcutaneous nodules that often ulcerate and drain, 4–6 weeks after exposure, often without a history of trauma.

Many environmental bacteria produce non-specific disease in humans: *MAIS*, *M. kansasii*, *M. malmoense*, *M. scrofulaceum*, *M. simiae*, *M. szulgai*, *M. xenopi*, *M. fortuitum*, *M. chelonae*[1]. Some environmental mycobacteria rarely produce disease in humans: *M. asiaticum*, *M. flavescens*, *M. gordonae*, *M. haemophilum*, *M. shimoidei*, *M. terrae*, *M. thermoresistibile*[1]. *M. malmoense* is primarily a pulmonary pathogen and *M. haemophilum* is primarily a cutaneous pathogen in immunocompromised patients. Regardless of the organism and the affected site, environmental mycobacteria frequently produce disease, especially pulmonary and cutaneous disease, that often resembles tuberculosis.

Two species of environmental mycobacteria, *M. marinum* and *M. ulcerans*, produce characteristic and distinctive skin disease, termed 'swimming pool' or 'fish tank granuloma' and 'Buruli ulcer' respectively. Such skin disease is invariably the result of inoculation from an exogenous source[11]. These two organisms and *M. fortuitum* and *M. chelonae* are the primary cutaneous pathogens that are currently responsible for the majority of skin disease produced by the environmental mycobacteria.

M. MARINUM

M. marinum is a slow growing environmental mycobacterium that produces characteristic and distinctive skin disease. Infection with *M. marinum* requires trauma, e.g. a cut, abrasion, scratch, etc., usually followed by exposure to the organism in a wet environment. Rivers, lakes, beaches, pools, swimming pools, etc. are common sources for infection, with either fresh or salt water. Sphagnum bogs are a particularly rich source for *M. marinum*[12]. The term 'swimming pool granuloma' applies to *M. marinum* skin disease that develops in this manner. The term 'fish tank granuloma' applies to the same disease produced by the same organism after exposure to the water or contents of a fish tank. 'Fish handler's granuloma' or 'fish fancier's granuloma' occurs in people who regularly handle fish via catching, cleaning, marketing, etc. In Japan approximately one-half of all reported cases of *M. marinum* skin disease are occupationally related to fish handling[13]; most of the other half of reported cases occur in fish tank hobbyists[13].

After inoculation of traumatized skin with the organism, a nondescript papule usually develops within 4–6 weeks over a bony surface. The papule enlarges to become a nodule or plaque, which often ulcerates (Figure 4.1). Occasionally plaques are warty or hyperkeratotic and may itch. Plaques or nodules are usually solitary[14] and the disease is usually unilateral, i.e. only one affected extremity (e.g. hand, foot, elbow, etc.)[13]. Frequently the plaques or nodules assume

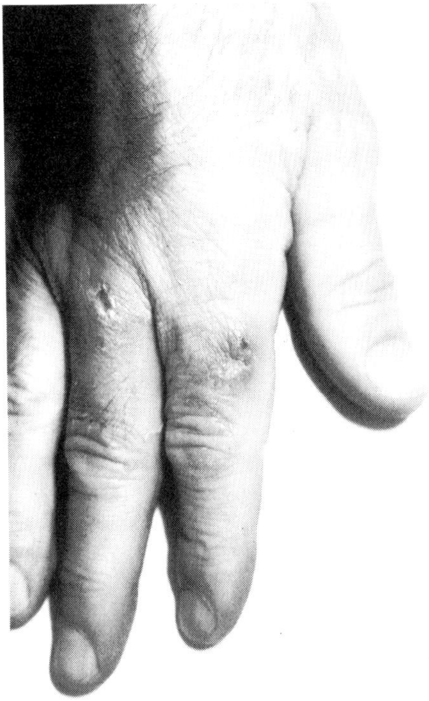

FIGURE 4.1 Ill-defined hyperkeratotic plaque on the hand, secondary to *M. marinum* infection acquired from a fish tank

a sporotrichoid appearance on the affected extremity[11,13–15] and may actually mimic sporotrichosis[13,16]. Skin disease heals with scarring. The most commonly affected site is the hand; other common sites are the knees and elbows, easily traumatized sites, especially in children while swimming. Tenosynovitis may accompany or precede skin disease[16]. Lymphadenopathy may occur but disseminated disease is very rare[11,16]. Eighty percent of affected patients have a positive PPD[11].

The differential diagnosis for *M. marinum* skin disease should include: warts, actinic and seborrhoeic keratoses, psoriasis, lichen planus, sporotrichosis, tuberculosis, blastomycosis, squamous cell carcinoma and Bowen's disease. History and morphology should suggest the correct diagnosis. Biopsy of a plaque or nodule is important and reveals a range of changes[17] – non-specific inflammation with suppuration in early stages and typical well-formed, non-caseating granulomas with the presence of acid-fast bacilli, usually few in number, in later stages. Histological changes may resemble those seen in tuberculosis verrucosa cutis or lupus vulgaris[16]. To establish the diagnosis, culture of tissue at 30°C is essential[17]. *M. marinum* is a photochromogen that grows well on Löwenstein–Jensen media at 30–32°C. The nitrate reduction test is a confirmatory biochemical test that is negative for *M. marinum* in contrast to *M. tuberculosis* and *M. kansasii*, for which the test is positive.

Treatment for *M. marinum* skin disease varies and depends primarily on the extent of disease. For isolated plaques or nodules, excision is preferable. Other reasonable approaches to the treatment of localized disease include: cryotherapy, curettage or heat. If several plaques or nodules are present or if skin disease affects a large area, chemotherapy is usually necessary, and should involve one of the following approaches: tetracycline[18] or minocycline[6,13] or doxycycline[6], all in high doses; the combination of trimethoprim and sulphamethoxazole[6,14]; or the combination of rifampin and ethambutol[6,14,19–21]. Each approach has provided good results in most patients. Cycloserine and ethionamide may be helpful as alternative drugs. Infection with *M. marinum* does not require drug susceptibility testing[6], since there is little evidence of resistance to this organism when tested against standard agents. For some patients treatment may not be necessary since *M. marinum* infection usually resolves; disease may persist for 2–3 years[11]. Nevertheless, treatment for either localized or extensive skin disease is usually reasonable and necessary. Human infection does not provide immunity from subsequent infection and BCG does not provide protection from infection.

M. FORTUITUM AND *M. CHELONAE*

M. fortuitum and M. chelonae are distinct and separate species with five sub-groups that produce non-descript subcutaneous and cutaneous disease, invariably as soft tissue abscesses and wound infections that usually follow trauma or surgery and often escape accurate diagnosis. Wound infections account for approximately 50% of all infections with these organisms. Found in soil and water, the organisms are facultative, nosocomial pathogens of increasing importance; compared to *M. tuberculosis* they are weak pathogens. The organisms can produce a wide spectrum of clinical disease[22], including non-cavitary pneumonia, endocarditis, lymphadenitis, osteomyelitis and keratitis. Skin disease, often hospital-acquired, follows injection, penetrating trauma[22,23], or surgery. Augmentation mammoplasty[22] and heart surgery[22] are two procedures that commonly precede wound infections, which are usually peri-prosthetic and refractory to treatment[24]. With such infections there was no evidence of a common contaminated product[24]. *M. chelonae* has produced wound infections after plastic surgery that involved the use of contaminated gentian violet as a skin marking solution[25] as well as wound infections in renal dialysis patients[9].

After inoculation of the organism into the skin or subcutaneous tissue, a cellulitis, nondescript abscess, nodule or group of nodules develops within 4–6 weeks at or adjacent to the site of the wound. The nodules or abscess usually drain serosanguinous or purulent material[24] and may produce sinus tracts (Figure 4.2). Commonly affected sites are: leg and foot, after injury; thigh, after injection; and trunk, after surgery[22]. Affected patients are usually afebrile and asymptomatic and have a negative PPD, in contrast to those patients affected with *M. marinum*. Disseminated disease is rare and mortality is low[7]; in contrast, morbidity may be significant. Cutaneous and subcutaneous skin disease heals with prominent scarring. The pathology of the affected tissue is usually non-specific. To establish an accurate diagnosis, culture, preferably of tissue, is necessary.

Excision with extensive debridement is the best form of treatment for localized disease[23]. For extensive or chronic disease, most patients require surgery with or without chemotherapy[26], dependent on *in vitro* drug sensitivity. Unfortunately, *M. fortuitum* and *M. chelonae* are notoriously resistant to antituberculous drugs[19], but do show some sensitivity to several antibiotics. The best drugs for *M. fortuitum* are amikacin or amikacin and cefoxitin, followed by a sulphonamide[26]; for *M. chelonae* the best drugs are amikacin or erythromycin or doxycycline or cefoxitin or amikacin and cefoxitin[26]. These agents have provided a good response and very few relapses in affected patients. Other studies have indicated benefits from cefoxitin and occasionally sulphonamides[7] and doxycycline and amikacin, combined with a sulphonamide and/or erythromycin[19].

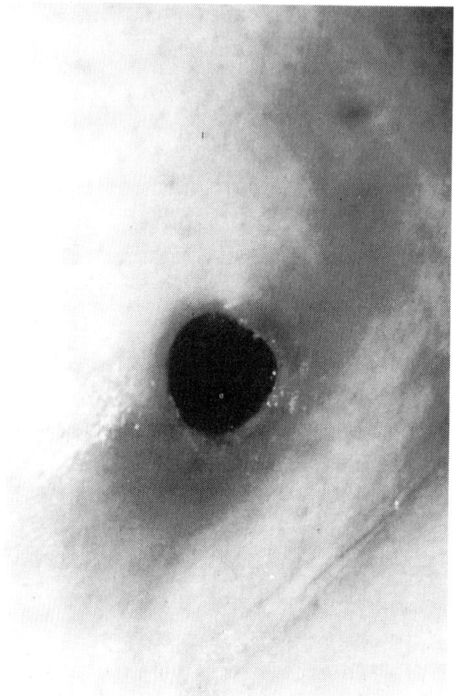

FIGURE 4.2 Draining abscess with surrounding cellulitis on the chest wall, secondary to *M. fortuitum* infection after mammoplasty

M. ULCERANS

M. ulcerans is an important environmental mycobacterium most commonly found in Africa and Australia. The organism is very rare in other parts of the world except for isolated reports usually as a result of travel to endemic areas. Exclusive of tuberculosis and leprosy, *M. ulcerans* is probably the most common cause of mycobacterial disease in humans[12].

Initially termed the 'Bairnsdale ulcer', based on the first description of disease in 1948 from the Bairnsdale area of Australia, a similar but supposedly unrelated disease occurred a few years later in the Buruli district of Uganda and received the label 'Buruli ulcer'. The same organism is now the accepted cause for both diseases with 'Buruli ulcer' as the accepted name for skin disease produced by *M. ulcerans*.

Similar cases have occurred in koalas, without any evidence of the transmission of the disease between koalas and humans[27].

Infection with *M. ulcerans* is most common in Africa and certain parts of Australia; it mainly affects children[28]. Infection is often seasonal, usually in the autumn and winter[27] and usually occurs in wet flooded marshy areas. Minor trauma, usually to an exposed surface, precedes most infections; disease requires environmental contact. Nonetheless, there is no report of isolation of the organism from the environment. The most commonly affected site is the leg. Disease begins with painless subcutaneous swelling, later with lateral and vertical extension to produce fasciitis, and finally ulceration that may produce large disfiguring defects that can involve an entire extremity. Despite extensive and necrotic disease, patients are asymptomatic and the need for hospitalization is minimal. Healing occurs with prominent scarring and often pronounced contracture, especially when large surface areas are affected. The skin test to Buruli extract is negative in the ulcerative or anergic phase of the disease, but later becomes positive when cellular immunity returns. Skin tests are often valuable in the absence of unavailable histological and microbiological information[27]. Representative pathology from a biopsy of an ulcer edge reveals numerous acid-fast bacilli in the ulcerative or anergic phase and typical non-caseating granulomas in later stages when cellular immunity returns. Biopsy and culture help to confirm the diagnosis; often these measures are not possible and often unnecessary in those endemic areas where the disease is common and well known to patients and physicians.

M. ulcerans grows easily on Löwenstein–Jensen media at 30–32°C. It is a non-chromogenic, slow growing mycobacterium that yields negative reactions to most of the standard biochemical tests used to identify other mycobacteria. By strict criteria, *M. ulcerans* is not part of the Runyon classification.

Therapy for this disease is challenging and demanding. Wide excision and grafting are still the best treatment[4]. Patient education in endemic areas is very important, helps to identify disease early and allows easier treatment. With extensive or ill-defined disease, wide excision and extensive grafting are often necessary, combined with physiotherapy and antituberculous drugs, even though none of the available drugs has shown much benefit.

CONCLUSION

The environmental mycobacteria are important organisms capable of producing a wide spectrum of human disease. Infections now occur with increased frequency and can pose significant problems in diagnosis and treatment. The main pathogens of the skin, *M. marinum*, *M. ulcerans*, *M. fortuitum* and *M. chelonae*, deserve the respect of dermatologists and other physicians who treat skin disease.

ACKNOWLEDGEMENTS

I want to thank my wife, Eileen, for her support and encouragement, and Carole Mays Kennedy for her suggestions and assistance.

REFERENCES

1. Grange, J. M. (1987). Infection and disease due to the environmental mycobacteria. *Trans. R. Soc. Trop. Med. Hyg.*, **81,** 179–82
2. Stine, T. M., Harris, A. A., Levin, S., Rivera, N. and Kaplan, R. L. (1987). A pseudoepidemic due to atypical mycobacteria in a hospital water supply. *J. Am. Med. Assoc.*, **258,** 809–11
3. Editorial (1981). Opportunistic mycobacteria. *Lancet,* **1,** 424
4. Wolinsky, E. (1979). Nontuberculous mycobacteria and associated diseases. *Am. Rev. Resp. Dis.*, **119,** 107–59
5. Runyon, E. H. (1959). Anonymous mycobacteria in pulmonary disease. *Med. Clin. N. Am.*, **43,** 273–90
6. Wallace, R. J., Jr. (1987). Recent clinical advances in knowledge of the nonleprous environmental mycobacteria responsible for cutaneous disease. (editorial). *Arch. Dermatol.*, **123,** 337–9
7. Brown, T. H. (1985). The rapidly growing mycobacteria – *Mycobacterium fortuitum* and *Mycobacterium chelonei. Infect. Control,* **6,** 283–8
8. Wickman, K. (1986). Clinical significance of nontuberculous mycobacteria. *Scand. J. Infect. Dis.*, **18,** 337–45
9. Woods, G. L. and Washington, J. A. II (1987). Mycobacteria other than *Mycobacterium tuberculosis:* review of microbiologic and clinical aspects. *Rev. Infect. Dis.*, **9,** 275–94
10. Young, L. S., Inderlied, C. B., Berlin, O. G. and Gottlieb, M. S. (1986). Mycobacterial infections in AIDS patients, with an emphasis on the *Mycobacterium avium* complex. *Rev. Infect. Dis.*, **8,** 1024–33
11. Beyt, B. E., Jr., Ortbals, D. W., Santa Cruz, D. J., Kobayashi, G. S., Eisen, A. Z. and Medoff, G. (1980). Cutaneous mycobacteriosis: analysis of 34 cases with a new classification of the disease. *Medicine,* **60,** 95–109

12. Grange, J. M. (1982). Mycobacteria and the skin. *Intern. J. Dermatol.*, **21,** 497–503
13. Arai, H., Nakajima, H. and Nagai, R. (1984). *Mycobacterium marinum* infection of the skin in Japan. *J. Dermatol.*, **11,** 37–42
14. Huminer, D., Pitlik, S. D., Block, C., Kaufman, L., Amit, S. and Rosenfeld, J. B. (1986). Aquarium-borne *Mycobacterium marinum* skin infection. *Arch. Dermatol.*, **122,** 698–703
15. Raz, I., Katz, M., Aram, H. and Haas, H. (1984). Sporotrichoid *Mycobacterium marinum* infection. *Intern. J. Dermatol.*, **23,** 554–5
16. Prevost, E., Walker, E. M. Jr., Kreutner, A. Jr. and Manos, J. (1982). *Mycobacterium marinum* infections: diagnosis and treatment. *South Med. J.*, **75,** 1349–52
17. Travis, W. D., Travis, L. B., Roberts, G. D., Su, D. W. and Weiland, L. W. (1985). The histopathologic spectrum in *Mycobacterium marinum* infection. *Arch. Pathol. Lab. Med.*, **109,** 1109–13
18. Hurst, L. C., Amadio, P. C., Badalamente, M. A., Ellstein, J. L. and Dattwyler, R. J. (1987). *Mycobacterium marinum* infections of the hand. *J. Hand Surg.*, **12A,** 428–35
19. Bass, J. B. Jr. and Hawkins, E. L. (1983). Treatment of disease caused by non-tuberculous mycobacteria. *Arch. Intern. Med.*, **143,** 1439–41
20. Donta, S. T., Smith, P. W., Levitz, R. E. and Quintiliani, R. (1986). Therapy of *Mycobacterium marinum* infections. *Arch. Intern. Med.*, **146,** 902–4
21. Brown, J. W., III and Sanders, C. V. (1987). *Mycobacterium marinum* infections. A problem of recognition, not therapy? (editorial) *Arch. Intern. Med.*, **147,** 817–18
22. Wallace, R. J., Jr., Swenson, J. M., Silcox, V. A., Good, R. C., Tschen, J. A. and Seabury Stone, M. (1983). Spectrum of disease due to rapidly growing mycobacteria. *Rev. Infect. Dis.*, **5,** 657–79
23. Kanta Subbarao, E., Tarpay, M. M. and Marks, M. I. (1987). Soft-tissue infections caused by *Mycobacterium fortuitum* complex following penetrating injury. *AJDC*, **141,** 1018–20
24. Clegg, H. W., Foster, M. T., Sanders, W. E., Jr. and Blaine, W. B. (1983). Infection due to organisms of the *Mycobacterium fortuitum* complex after augmentation mammaplasty: clinical and epidemiologic features. *J. Infect. Dis.*, **147,** 427–33
25. Safranek, T. J., Jarvis, W. R., Carson, L. A., Cusick, L. B., Bland, L. E., Swenson, J. M. and Silcox, V. A. (1987). *Mycobacterium chelonae* wound infections after plastic surgery employing contaminated gentian violet skin-marking solution. *N. Engl. J. Med.*, **317,** 197–201
26. Wallace, R. J. Jr., Swenson, J. M., Silcox, V. A. and Bullen, M. G. (1985). Treatment of nonpulmonary infections due to *Mycobacterium fortuitum* and *Mycobacterium chelonei* on the basis of *in vitro* susceptibilities. *J. Infect. Dis.*, **152,** 500–14
27. Hayman, J. (1985). Clinical features of *Mycobacterium ulcerans* infection. *Aust. J. Dermatol.*, **26,** 67–73
28. Burchard, G. D. and Bierther, M. (1986). Buruli ulcer: clinical pathological study of 23 patients in Lambarene, Gabon. *Trop. Med. Parasit.*, **37,** 1–8

5

LEPROSY: CLINICAL ASPECTS

A. C. McDOUGALL

The World Health Organization (WHO) Expert Committee on Leprosy has recently confirmed[1] that the world prevalence is between 10 and 12 million cases, with more than 1.6 billion people living in countries where the estimated prevalence is greater than one case per 1000 population. The main leprosy endemic areas are in South and Central America and Mexico; Africa, India and the Far East. In the past 20 years, there has been a steady increase in the number of cases registered, reaching 5.4 million in 1985, a figure which represents a 90% increase over that for 1966. The total number in 1987 was 5.1 million, a drop which has been interpreted[2] as at least partly due to the implementation of WHO recommendations on multiple drug therapy[3], with release from treatment of considerable numbers of patients. Despite impressive progress in microbiology, immunology and molecular biology in recent years, with the possibility of developing a vaccine against leprosy, together with serological tests which may be of value in diagnosis, classification and management[4], the cornerstone of our approach to the management of individual cases and the control of leprosy rests firmly on case detection and treatment with multiple drug combinations. Much of this chapter will give emphasis to those aspects of leprosy which have a direct practical bearing on the wider implementation of multiple drug therapy (hereafter MDT) as recommended by WHO in 1982[3].

DIAGNOSIS

The diagnosis of leprosy may be based on either clinical findings, microscopic findings or examination of slit-skin smears, or histopathological findings in a biopsy, or a combination of all three. Other potentially valuable diagnostic procedures, mainly involving serological tests, are under development[4], but not yet generally available. With regard to clinical findings, pure observation, coupled with experience of the various forms of leprosy (described below) as seen on the skin or found on examination of peripheral nerves, goes a long way towards establishing the diagnosis in many cases (Figures 5.1 and 5.2). There is, however, no short-cut to the acquisition of skills in the recognition of the varied and at times perplexing manifestations of this disease on the skin, including ability to detect the subtle changes in pigmentation and texture which indicate an early lesion. Particularly for those whose background is in dermatology or other disciplines, it is sometimes difficult to appreciate the great importance of a detailed examination of the peripheral nerves in diagnosing and classifying leprosy. This calls for a basic knowledge of their anatomical course and function; an appreciation of those nerves relevant to leprosy which are (1) normally palpable in healthy individuals, and (2) *not* normally palpable (and are therefore abnormal if they can be palpated); and an ability to accurately compare the size and consistence of nerves on both sides of the body. The finding of a definitely enlarged nerve (Figure 5.3) even if not obviously associated with skin lesions, and especially if there are motor and/or sensory disturbances in its area of supply, is highly suggestive of leprosy and often diagnostic; there are extremely few other causes of enlargement of peripheral nerves in the field of clinical medicine (or neurology). It is important to recognize that the diagnosis of leprosy can, in fact, be established with confidence in a high percentage of cases on purely clinical grounds, though the addition of examination of slit-skin smears is preferable, *if properly performed.* The examination of slit-skin smears from lesions and/or routine sites is described in detail in standard books of reference[5–7]. Although a relatively simple technique, experience has however shown (as also in the case of sputum examination for tuberculosis) that the quality of performance frequently falls far below acceptable levels. Two recent publications[8,9] have drawn attention to what is generally

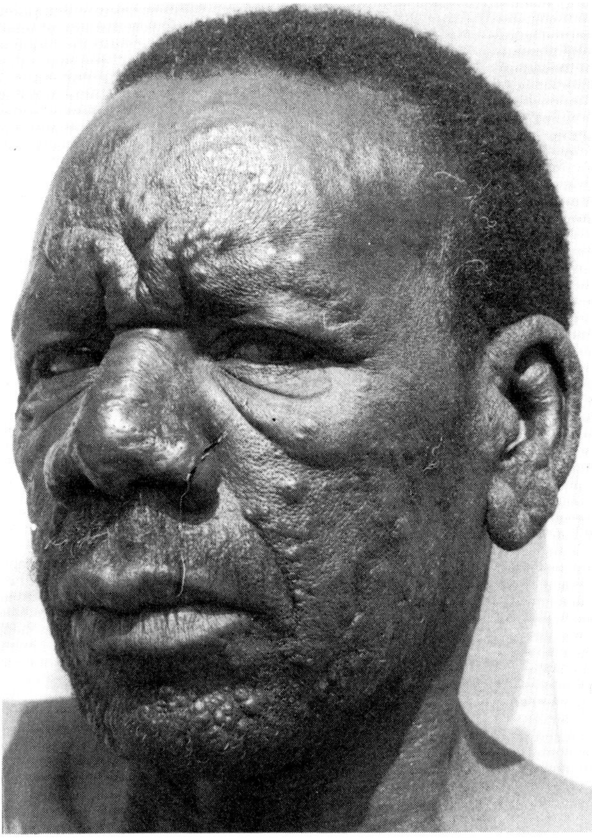

FIGURE 5.1 Lepromatous (LL) leprosy of several years duration; thickening of the facial tissues, numerous bilateral symmetrical nodules, heavy involvement of the ears, loss of eyelashes and eyebrows (madarosis). Skin smears and nasal mucus highly positive for acid-fast bacilli

an unsatisfactory and even hazardous state of affairs in many control programmes and hospital laboratories, with a strong plea for the establishment, at least at the outset, of one centre of excellence, where results are completely *reliable*. In cases of doubt, clinical judgement, based on experience, should always take precedence over a laboratory report of questionable accuracy in the diagnosis of leprosy.

Biopsy of skin (less commonly of other tissues) is a valuable procedure in some circumstances, but not absolutely essential in the

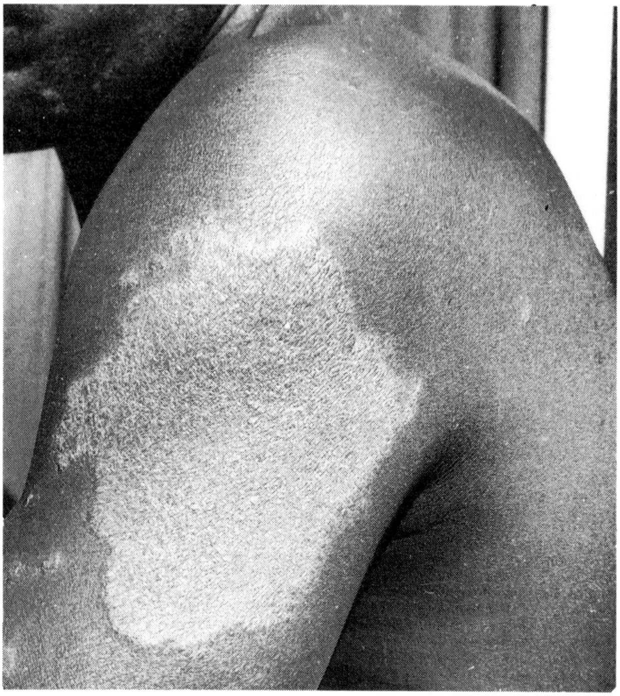

FIGURE 5.2 Tuberculoid (TT) leprosy. This large patch on the deltoid region was dry, non-sweating and totally devoid of sensation on testing with cotton wool, pin prick and hot and cold tubes. Skin smears were completely negative for acid-fast bacilli

management of the individual case and positively inadvisable, for routine purposes, in control programmes. The taking, fixation, processing, microscopic examination and interpretation of biopsies in leprosy has been described in full by Ridley[10,11]. The procedure should be carried out only by medically qualified staff, with attention, notably in Africa and South America, to the possible risks related to HIV (and hepatitis B) infection, for which guidelines have been established by WHO[12]. Attention to technique is important; (1) the biopsy must be of full depth in order to include lower or subdermal nerves; (2) fixation must be good if the tissue is to be processed, cut and stained properly. Formol–Zenker solutions give best results, but for routine purposes 10% formalin is adequate, provided it is buffered and freshly made up. A well chosen skin biopsy, accompanied by clinical details and

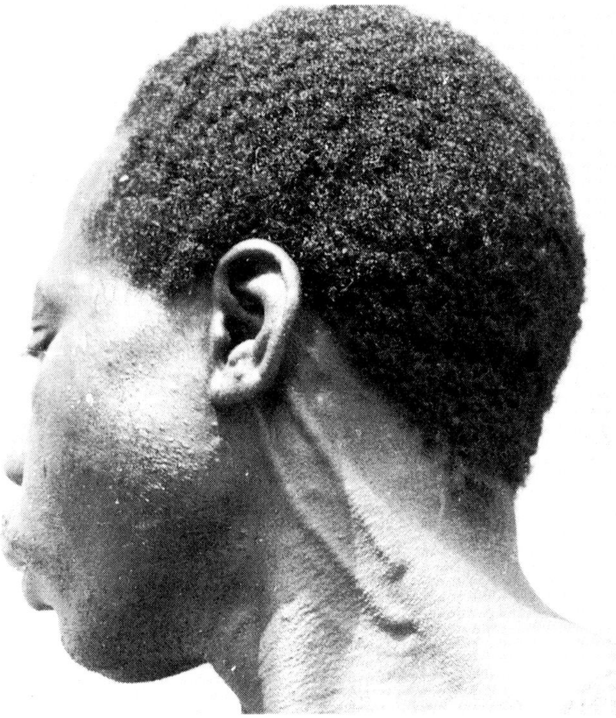

FIGURE 5.3 Markedly enlarged (duplicate branches) of the great auricular nerve in the neck. The original classification was borderline-tuberculoid (BT) leprosy, but by the time this photograph was taken, skin lesions were in fact impossible to see. There was loss of sensation in the skin over the parotid gland and at the back of the ear. Skin smears were negative from all sites

including an account of past and present drug treatment, can be of considerable value in difficult, individual cases, not only for diagnosis and classification, but also in attempting to distinguish between reactional states (see below) and relapse. Biopsies are essential in drug trials and other research projects before and during the course of any intervention. A biopsy of nerve may be indicated for diagnosis or classification, but should be performed only by an experienced, medically qualified operator, and only on nerves which are purely sensory (i.e. never on a peripheral nerve containing motor fibres).

In summary, the diagnosis of leprosy should rest mainly on observation, clinical examination of the entire body surface in a good light, palpation of peripheral nerves and testing for diminution or loss of sensation. If available *and reliable,* slit-skin smears should be performed and the results taken into consideration. In individual cases of doubt or difficulty, biopsy may be of further help. The lepromin test, using a standardized, autoclaved suspension of leprosy bacilli of either human or armadillo origin, for intradermal injection and reading 3–4 weeks later, is useful in classification (see below), but of no value in diagnosis. Finally, it is useful to recognize that the diagnosis of this disease is (1) not always easy, and (2) sometimes attended by considerable social and psychological upset. It should therefore be made with care and in cases of doubt there should be no hesitation in referring cases to an experienced observer. Newcomers to endemic areas, whether medically qualified or not, would do well to remember that indigenous paramedical staff, with long experience of control programmes, may be invaluable in this context.

CLASSIFICATION

From a clinical point of view, leprosy is a complex disease with a remarkable range of manifestations in both skin and peripheral nerves. The earlier systems of classification referred almost entirely to clinical findings such as nodules, plaques, anaesthesia, etc., but there gradually evolved, from workers in South America, Europe and India, the concept of a disease with a spectrum of response related to the immunological capacity of the individual. One of the most highly developed of these is the Ridley–Jopling 'System of classification of leprosy according to immunity', published in 1966[13] and now widely accepted, not only for research purposes, but also for clinical use and control programmes. It is based on a closely observed association between clinical findings in skin and nerve, slit-skin smears, biopsies and lepromin test. The main features of this comprehensive and valuable system are shown in Table 5.1. It is worth noting that the spectrum does not represent a continuous 'sliding' scale, but that each type of leprosy (TT, BT, etc.) has its own well-defined characteristics, with a good correlation between clinical and histopathological findings. The other systems, including a number from South America, the Madrid classification and various modifications from India are to a considerable

TABLE 5.1 The Ridley–Jopling classification

Type of leprosy	*Symbol*	*Level (strength) CMI**	*Lepromin test*	*Acid-fast bacilli in lesions*	*Sensation in skin lesions*	*Grouping for the purpose of multidrug therapy (MDT) as advised by WHO*
Tuberculoid	TT	+ + + +	strongly positive	none (or extremely few)	absent	paucibacillary (PB)
Borderline tuberculoid	BT	+ +/+ + +	weakly positive	none or scanty	moderately diminished	paucibacillary (PB)
Midborderline	BB	+ +	negative	moderate numbers	moderate to slight diminution	multibacillary (MB)
Borderline-lepromatous	BL	+	negative	many	slight diminution	multibacillary (MB)
Lepromatous	LL	0	negative	very numerous	not affected	multibacillary (MB)

* Arbitrary '+' units for the purpose of this table only

extent embraced in the Ridley–Jopling system, which is probably now the most frequently used for the grouping of patients into either pauci- or multibacillary forms of leprosy for the purposes of multiple drug therapy (MDT) as recommended by WHO in 1982[3]. Terminology has, understandably, given rise to much argument through the decades, but it is no longer a serious obstacle and the need to classify cases has focused attention on the practical relevance of classification for treatment purposes. It has, of course, also a bearing on prognosis, the total duration of treatment, the follow-up needed, the type of management which may be required, and the possible risks of infection to family and immediate contacts.

Three additional forms of leprosy, not included in the above system, require further description.

Indeterminate leprosy

This is a relatively early form of the disease, in which the outcome is 'undetermined', usually manifesting as one, or a very few, flat (macular) lesions; hypopigmented or erythematous; often with ill-defined margins. Slit-skin smears are usually negative for bacilli. A well taken, full-depth skin biopsy may reveal a round-cell infiltrate in or around appendages and along neurovascular pathways, possibly including invasion of nerve and the finding of bacilli in nerve – but this is unusual; more often skin biopsy is either negative or unhelpful. This type of leprosy may disappear spontaneously or persist for long periods, or develop into one of the 'determined forms' of leprosy. For the purpose of MDT, it is included in the paucibacillary (PB) group.

Neural or 'pure' neural leprosy

Particularly from India (and much less commonly from other parts of the world), a form of leprosy has been described in which there is involvement of one or more peripheral nerves, but without any skin lesions. Many of these cases have been proven on nerve biopsy, which also reveals the classification to be usually in the TT–BT range. A lepromin test may also be of value in establishing a classification. Particularly in countries other than India, it is, however, important before making a diagnosis of neural leprosy to be quite sure that no skin lesions can be seen on any part of the body, after full examination of the entire skin surface in a good light. It has also to be remembered that skin lesions, following adequate chemotherapy, may disappear, but that neural manifestations may remain. The opinion of an experienced observer may be invaluable.

Lucio leprosy

This is an unusual form of leprosy, mainly confined to Mexico, but occasionally reported from other areas. It has been reviewed in detail by Frenken[14]. There is a diffuse, non-nodular infiltration of the skin, with loss of body hair, including eyebrows and eyelashes (but not the hair of the scalp), together with widespread sensory loss due to involvement of dermal nerves. Bacilli are present in all parts of the skin in large numbers and treatment is essentially as for lepromatous (LL) leprosy.

REACTIONS ('REACTIONAL STATES')

Apart from the basic forms of leprosy described above, it has to be recognized that leprosy is characterized by phenomena which, although apparently mainly clinical, have underlying immunological changes, related to either humoral or cell-mediated immune mechanisms. The commonly encountered reactions can be divided, with fair accuracy, into those towards the lepromatous end of the spectrum which are dependent upon humoral (immune-complex) factors and those in other parts of the spectrum, which are dependent on cell-mediated immune (CMI) factors. Jopling has divided reactions or 'reactional states' into Types 1 and 2[15]. Type 1 reactions depend on cell-mediated immune (CMI) factors and delayed hypersensitivity (corresponding to Coombs and Gell Type IV) and they occur predominantly in borderline (dimorphous) patients. There are often rapid changes in CMI, accompanied by striking clinical changes.

If there is an *increase* in CMI, as seen not uncommonly in patients on treatment, the reaction is referred to as 'reversal' (*syn.* upgrading). If the reaction is associated with a *reduction* in immunity, the reaction is termed 'downgrading'. Clinically, there is a rapid change in the appearance of some or all of the lesions which become red, raised and occasionally ulcerate. Nerve involvement is common and may result in catastrophically sudden and serious damage to motor and sensory axons. In Type 2 reaction, there is no significant change in CMI and the changes are those of an immune-complex syndrome involving antigen, antibody and complement, corresponding to Type III (Coombs and Gell). It occurs almost exclusively in lepromatous (LL) leprosy. The basic leprosy lesions do not change, but crops of new lesions in the form of red or dusky red nodules appear on the arms, legs and face, less commonly on other parts of the body. The patient has systemic upset with fever, joint pains, malaise, loss of weight, neuritis, lymphadenitis, iritis, orchitis and proteinuria. Detailed descriptions of both these types of reaction may be found in standard works[16–18], but for the purpose of this chapter the most important point to make is that reactions in leprosy are part and parcel of the day-to-day management of patients, with an appreciable incidence in both pauci- and multibacillary cases in most parts of the world. Their importance cannot be overstated, since nerve damage during the course of both types of reaction is common, affecting both motor and sensory elements, and is a major cause of disability and deformity. It is remarkable and highly regrettable that we know very little of the underlying mechanisms and still less about precipitating factors for reactions in leprosy – but encouraging to note that the Special Programme for Research and Training in Tropical Diseases (TDR) has recently given high priority to basic research to resolve this problem. Although treatment is available for both Type 1 and Type 2 reactions, the drugs used (steroids, clofazimine and thalidomide) are by no means without complications and side-effects and in practice, under programme conditions in third world countries, it is not easy to ensure that patients in danger of nerve damage receive medication early and regularly. It would be of the greatest help to be able to predict those patients or even the circumstances, in which reactions are particularly likely to occur, and it is to be hoped that systematic attention will be given to such research as a matter of urgency. Before leaving the subject of diagnosis, classification and reactions, some thought has to be given to the possible impact of the acquired immunodeficiency syndrome (AIDS) on leprosy. The already well-documented evidence for both a clinical and epidemiological association between AIDS and tuberculosis has recently been reviewed by Nunn and McAdam[19] and they also discuss the possible effect that AIDS may have on clinical findings and reactional states in leprosy. There is, in fact, no documented evidence so far for a significant association between AIDS and leprosy, but the possibility that this immunodepressant viral infection may alter the clinical picture, response to treatment and the pattern of reaction in leprosy, has clearly to be kept in mind. It has also to be envisaged, perhaps particularly in Africa and South America, that the financial and professional burden of AIDS may divert resources from the control of other communicable diseases, including leprosy.

DISABILITY AND DEFORMITY IN LEPROSY

Of the 5.1 million patients reported by WHO[1] to be currently registered, about 30% have significant disabilities and the same percentage may be expected from the total of 10–12 million estimated to have leprosy. It bears repetition that the effect of leprosy on nerves, leading to paralysis or anaesthesia, is by far the most important. Skin lesions are arresting, often lead to presentation and diagnosis, but they disappear in many instances with good chemotherapy and are rarely of long-term significance. Nerve damage, by contrast, may be not only extensive but also irreversible, especially in situations where facilities do not exist within reasonable distance of the patient's home, for expert care. Running through the entire subject of leprosy, including all the forms described above (except indeterminate) and the reactional states, there is therefore a disturbing element of disability and deformity which is of crucial importance to both individual patients and the success of control programmes. It is essential to do all possible to ensure that 'disability control' ranks side by side with 'bacillus control', using methodology and techniques which are both available and effective, if properly applied[20].

THE TREATMENT OF THE BACILLARY INFECTION IN LEPROSY

Dapsone was introduced in the 1940s and used as monotherapy for several decades. But, in the 1960s and 1970s, it became increasingly apparent that dapsone resistance was a widespread and increasing phenomenon[21]. This, perhaps, more than anything else stimulated WHO to convene a meeting of experts in 1981 and to publish in 1982 their recommendations: *Chemotherapy of leprosy for control programmes*[3], in which it was advised that all cases of leprosy, whatever the classification, should receive *multiple* drug treatment. For this purpose, WHO divided all cases into two groups: (1) multibacillary (MB) to include lepromatous (LL), borderline-lepromatous (BL) and mid-borderline (BB) on the Ridley–Jopling scale, and (2) paucibacillary (PB) to include tuberculoid (TT) and borderline-tuberculoid (BT) on the Ridley–Jopling Scale. Indeterminate (though not in the original Ridley–Jopling classification) is included in the paucibacillary group.

TABLE 5.2 Multiple drug regimens for pauci- and multibacillary leprosy patients (adult dose) (WHO; 'Chemotherapy of leprosy for control programmes'; Technical Report Series 675, 1982)

Multibacillary patients: (LL, BL and BB on the Ridley–Jopling Scale)
Monthly, supervised medication: – rifampicin 600 mg
– clofazimine 300 mg

Daily, unsupervised medication: – dapsone 100 mg
– clofazimine 50 mg

Duration: A minimum of 2 years but wherever possible until slit-skin smears are negative

Follow-up after stopping treatment: a minimum of 5 years, with clinical and bacteriological examination at least every 12 months

Paucibacillary patients (TT, BT on the Ridley–Jopling scale and Indeterminate)
Monthly, supervised medication: – rifampicin 600 mg

Daily, unsupervised medication: – dapsone 100 mg

Duration: 6 months; all treatment then stops

Follow-up after stopping treatment: a minimum of 2 years with clinical examination at least every 12 months

The drug regimens for adult patients are shown in Table 5.2, those for children in Tables 5.3 and 5.4. It is extremely encouraging to note that these regimens have now been implemented widely in various parts of the world with good results. They are acceptable to patients and staff, effective clinically and bacteriologically, capable of reducing disability rates, and are not attended by an undue incidence of toxic effects or relapse. But unfortunately the overall, worldwide rate of implementation and the number of patients so far covered have fallen short of expectations and there is an urgent need to define and correct the factors which are impeding the better use of a form of treatment which is available and manifestly effective. A considerable amount of interest has recently been shown in the use of blister-calendar packs for MDT in leprosy and Figures 5.4 and 5.5 carry diagrams similar to those which are already in widespread use in India, Thailand and the Philippines.

TABLE 5.3 Multiple drug regimens for paucibacillary leprosy (WHO, 1982) based on age of children (two drugs – dapsone and rifampicin). Where a range of doses is given this relates to age range of the children; those nearer the lower age range receive the lower dose and those near the upper age range receive the higher dose. (With acknowledgements to *Leprosy Review*, 1984, **55,** 309)

Age groups	*Dapsone: daily dose unsupervised*	*Rifampicin: monthly dose supervised*
⩽5 years	25 mg	150–300 mg
6–14 years	50–100 mg	300–450 mg
⩾15 years*	100 mg	600 mg

* i.e. use adult doses

TABLE 5.4 Multiple drug regimens for multibacillary leprosy (WHO, 1982) based on age of children (three drugs – dapsone, rifampicin and clofazimine). Where a range of doses is given this relates to age range of the children; those nearer the lower age range receive the lower dose and those near the upper age range receive the higher dose. (With acknowledgements to *Leprosy Review*, 1984, **55,** 309)

Age groups	*Dapsone: daily dose unsupervised*	*Clofazimine*		*Rifampicin monthly dose supervised*
		Unsupervised dose	*Monthly dose supervised*	
⩽5 years	25 mg	100 mg once weekly	100 mg	150–300 mg
6–14 years	50–100 mg	150 mg once weekly	150–200 mg	300–450 mg
⩾15 years	100 mg	50 mg daily	300 mg	600 mg

THE TREATMENT OF REACTIONS ('REACTIONAL STATES') IN LEPROSY

The approach is different for Type 1 and Type 2, as defined above. In the case of Type 1, reactions where the mechanisms are mainly concerned with CMI, moderate or severe reactions require treatment, more or less as a matter of urgency, with systemic steroids. Specialist texts should be consulted for details, but in general the adult dose required at the onset is often in the order of 30–40 mg prednisolone or equivalent per day. In practice it is often possible to halve the daily total dose within a few days, then reduce by about 10 mg weekly, finishing with 10 mg on alternate days until the reaction is controlled. There are, of course, well-known hazards to the use of steroids, especially in debilitated people in Third World countries, and some degree of expert supervision is to be preferred, including attention to risks of concomitant (and perhaps unrecognized) tuberculosis. Mild Type 1 reactions may respond quite well to aspirin or similar analgesics but it is important to be alert to the possibility of low-grade 'silent' neuritis[1] which may insidiously lead to irreversible damage, especially as there is evidence that it can be prevented by the judicious use of steroids over a period of several months.

In the case of Type 2 reactions, where the mechanism is essentially immune-complex-mediated, steroids are also valuable, but two other drugs have been used with considerable success. Clofazimine is useful not only for the treatment of the bacillary infection (see above), but also for the treatment or suppression of Type 2 reactions. However, its mode of onset is slow and doses in the order of 200–300 mg daily are required for the treatment of such reactions, giving an incidence of gastrointestinal side-effects and skin pigmentation, which is often unacceptable. An alternative, where national regulations allow its use, is thalidomide, which is given to adults in a dose of 400 mg daily until the reaction is under control, thereafter reducing gradually to 50 mg daily. It is absolutely contraindicated in premenopausal women. Although capable of causing peripheral neuritis, as a toxic effect, neither this nor any of its side-effects have, in fact, been found disadvantageous in the treatment of this form of reaction in leprosy. It is useless, and should not be used, for Type 1 reactions.

SOCIAL AND PSYCHOLOGICAL ASPECTS

No account of the treatment of this disease would be complete without a section drawing attention to the importance of social and psychological factors. This is a disturbing, at times frightening, disease; it is potentially disabling and often associated in the public mind with gross disfigurement and social upheaval. The fact that it can be treated

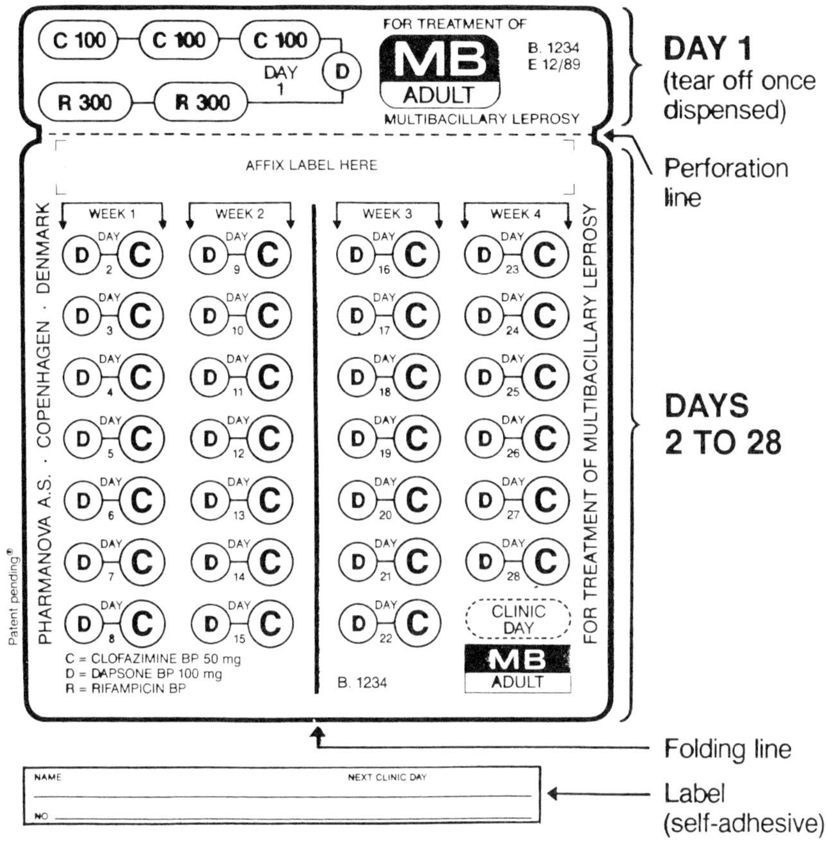

DAY 1	**Supervised** monthly dose.
DAYS 2 TO 28	**Self-administered** daily doses.
DAY 29	**Clinic day**

FIGURE 5.4 Diagram of a blister-calendar pack used for the triple drug treatment of patients with multibacillary (MB) leprosy. The upper detachable part carries the monthly supervised dose of rifampicin (600 mg) and clofazimine (300 mg), with a tablet of dapsone (100 mg). The remainder of the pack carries the daily, unsupervised doses of dapsone (100 mg) and clofazimine (50 mg)

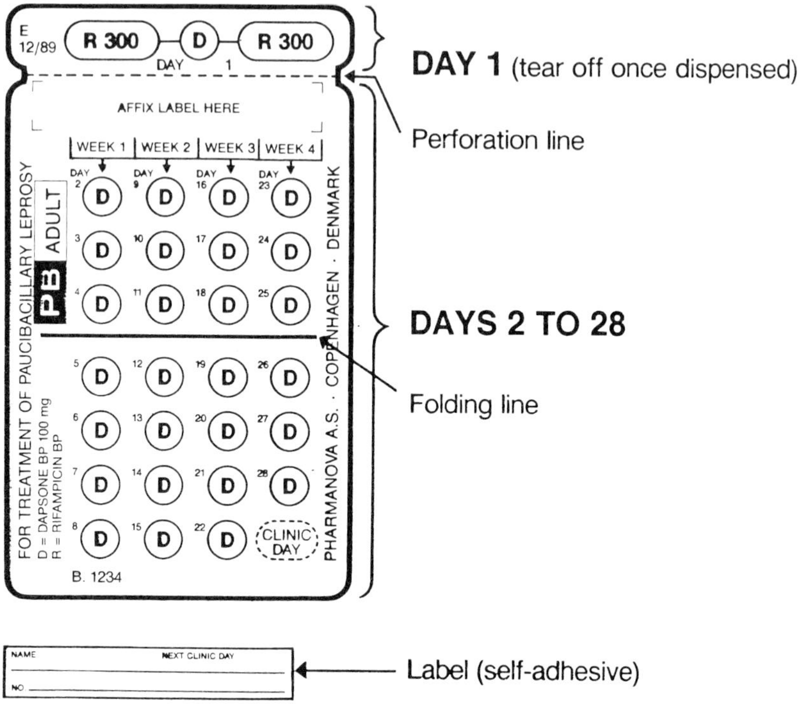

DAY 1	**Supervised** monthly dose.
DAYS 2 TO 28	**Self-administered** daily doses.
DAY 29	**Clinic day**

FIGURE 5.5 Diagram of a blister-calendar pack for the dual drug treatment of patients with paucibacillary (PB) leprosy. The upper detachable part carries the monthly, supervised dose of rifampicin (600 mg), with a tablet of dapsone (100 mg). The remainder of the pack carries the daily, unsupervised doses of dapsone (100 mg). (With acknowledgements to Pharmanova A.S., Copenhagen, Denmark)

with great success if diagnosed early and properly managed, on an outpatient basis, in well over 90% of all cases, is still poorly appreciated by millions of people in leprosy-endemic areas. At an individual level, careful explanation, patience and reassurance are often essential. Killing the bacilli is important; it must be done thoroughly and effectively, making the best use of the excellent drugs available. But the 'treatment' of the patient, in the fullest sense of the word, calls for much more, and a failure to address disability, fear, social and family aspects, loss of employment and self-respect, will have repercussions for both individuals and control programmes.

CONCLUSION

If these and other problems in the implementation of MDT can be overcome, and case-detection increased, preferably through integrated (general) health services, using the primary health care approach[22], the outlook for control of this disease is not only good, but almost certainly better now than at any time in the past. To quote Dr S. K. Noordeen, Chief, Leprosy, Division of Communicable Disease, WHO, Geneva[23], 'The opportunities to markedly reduce leprosy in the next decade are immense. It remains to be seen whether or not we make use of them, and whether or not leprosy will ultimately be eliminated as a public health problem as part of the overall goal of "Health for All by the Year 2000".'

REFERENCES

1. WHO (1988). WHO Expert Committee on Leprosy. Sixth Report. Technical Report Series 768. (Geneva: World Health Organization)
2. Lopez-Bravo, L. (1988). Global Review of Implementation of MDT (Multiple Drug Therapy). *Third Coordinating Meeting on Implementation of Multidrug Therapy in Leprosy Control,* The Hague, 13 September
3. WHO (1982) Chemotherapy of Leprosy for Control Programmes. Report of a WHO Study Group. Technical Report Series 675. (Geneva: World Health Organization)
4. UNDP/World Bank/WHO (1987). Tropical Diseases Research: A Global partnership. Report of the Special Programme for Research & Training in Tropical Diseases (TDR). (Geneva: World Health Organization)
5. Leiker, D. L. and McDougall, A. C. (1987). *Technical Guide for Smear Examination for Leprosy.* 2nd revised edn. (Wurzburg, Germany: Deutsches Aussätzigen Hilfswerke e.V.)
6. Cheesbrough, M. (1984). *Medical Laboratory Manual for Tropical Countries. Tropical Health Technology,* Vol. II. (Doddington, Cambridgeshire: Tropical Health Technology)
7. King, M. (1973). *A Medical Laboratory for Developing Countries.* (London: Oxford University Press)

8. Georgiev, G. D. and McDougall, A. C. (1988). Skin smears and bacterial index (BI) in multiple drug therapy leprosy control programmes: an unsatisfactory and potentially hazardous state of affairs. Correspondence. *Int. J. Lepr.*, **56,** 101–4
9. Georgiev, G. D. and McDougall, A. C. (1987). The bacterial examination of slit-skin smears in leprosy control programmes using multiple drug therapy: a plea for radical changes in current operational methodology. *Int. J. Lepr.*, **59,** 373–85
10. Ridley, D. S. (1985). *Skin Biopsy in Leprosy*. Documents Geigy. 2nd edn. (Basle, Switzerland: Ciba-Geigy Ltd)
11. Ridley, D. S. (1974). Histological classification and the immunological spectrum of leprosy. *Bull. WHO*, **51,** 451
12. WHO (1987). Guidelines for personnel involved in collection of skin smears in leprosy control programmes for the prevention and control of possible infection with HIV. WHO/CDS/LEP87.1 Rev. 1
13. Ridley, D. S. and Jopling, W. H. (1966). Classification of leprosy according to immunity. *Int. J. Lepr.*, **34,** 255–73
14. Frenken, J. H. (1963). *Diffuse Leprosy of Lucio and Latapi*. De Wit Inc. Oranjestad, Aruba, Netherlands, Antilles
15. Jopling, W. H. (1959). Reactional leprosy or leprosy in reaction. *Lepr. Rev.*, **30,** 194–6
16. Hastings, R. C. (ed.) (1985). *Leprosy. Medicine in the Tropics*. (Edinburgh, London, Melbourne & New York: Churchill Livingstone)
17. Jopling, W. H. and McDougall, A. C. (1988). *Handbook of Leprosy*. 4th edn. (Oxford: Heinemann Professional Publishing)
18. Bryceson, A. and Pfaltzgraff, R. E. (1979). *Leprosy. Medicine in the Tropics*. (Edinburgh, London & New York: Churchill Livingstone)
19. Nunn, P. P. and McAdam, K. P. W. J. (1988). Mycobacterial infections and AIDS. In Rees, R. J. W. (ed.) *Tuberculosis and Leprosy. Br. Med. Bull.*, **44,** 3
20. WHO (1987). Report of the consultation on disability prevention and rehabilitation in leprosy. Geneva 9–11 March. WHO/COS/LEP87.3
21. Baohong, J. I. (1985). Drug-resistance in leprosy – a review. *Lepr. Rev.*, **56,** 265–78
22. Feenstra, P. and Tadele Tedla (1988). A broader scope for leprosy control. *Wld. Hlth Forum*, **9,** 53–8
23. Noordeen, S. K. (1987). Global review of MDT implementation. Paper presented to *WHO/SEARO Inter-country Seminar on Implementation and Evaluation of Multidrug Therapy in Leprosy Control Programmes through Primary Health Care*, SEARO, New Delhi, 7–11 December

INDEX